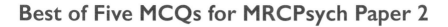

Best of Five MCQs for MRCPsych Paper 2

Best of Five MCQs for MRCPsych Paper 2

Lena Palaniyappan
Clinical Lecturer, Division of Psychiatry, University of Nottingham, Nottingham, UK

Rajeev Krishnadas
Clinical Lecturer, Sackler Institute of Psychobiological Research, University of Glasgow, Glasgow, UK

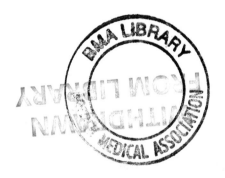

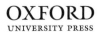

OXFORD
UNIVERSITY PRESS

OXFORD
UNIVERSITY PRESS

Great Clarendon Street, Oxford OX2 6DP

Oxford University Press is a department of the University of Oxford.
It furthers the University's objective of excellence in research, scholarship,
and education by publishing worldwide in

Oxford New York

Auckland Cape Town Dar es Salaam Hong Kong Karachi
Kuala Lumpur Madrid Melbourne Mexico City Nairobi
New Delhi Shanghai Taipei Toronto

With offices in

Argentina Austria Brazil Chile Czech Republic France Greece
Guatemala Hungary Italy Japan Poland Portugal Singapore
South Korea Switzerland Thailand Turkey Ukraine Vietnam

Oxford is a registered trade mark of Oxford University Press
in the UK and in certain other countries

Published in the United States
by Oxford University Press Inc., New York

British Library Cataloguing in Publication Data
Data available

Library of Congress Cataloguing in Publication Data
Data available

Typeset by Cepha Imaging Private Ltd., Bangalore, India
Printed in Great Britain
on acid-free paper by
Ashford Colour Press Limited, Gosport, Hampshire

ISBN 978–0–19–955212–2

10 9 8 7 6 5 4 3 2 1

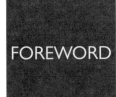

FOREWORD

Passing the MRCPsych examination is a major milestone in the career of every aspirant psychiatrist in the UK. This examination specifies the minimum levels of knowledge and skills that are essential for gaining the membership of the College.

Rajeev Krishnadas and Lena Palaniyappan have had extensive and varied training and experience, in both research and teaching. They are both clinical lecturers with proven track records in teaching, developing, and publishing educational materials and organizing the successful SPMM course for trainee psychiatrists. In fact, Lena Palaniyappan was awarded the Laughlin Prize in the MRCPsych exams.

There are many books of varying quality on the market for candidates sitting the MRCPsych exams. What differentiates an outstanding book from an ordinary book is that in addition to aiding passing the exams, the former also promotes learning that would ultimately make the readers wiser and help improve patient care.

The authors have used their teaching skills and experience to develop an exhaustive range of questions in the Royal College's new format. They have taken utmost care to perfectly match the questions with the Paper 2 syllabus, and to the levels of complexity and the topic-wise breakdown of questions in the real exams. They have organized the questions in five mutually exclusive chapters in a way that would facilitate focused learning. Finally, they provide detailed, well-researched and referenced explanatory answers for every question. Thus, they have made this a really outstanding book.

I recommend this excellent book to candidates sitting the Paper 2 of the MRCPsych examinations. I am confident that this book will significantly increase their chances of passing at the first attempt.

Albert Michael MBBS, DPM, MD, FRCPsych, FHEA
Organizer, Cambridge MRCPsych Course
Director of Medical Education, Suffolk Mental Health Trust
April 2009

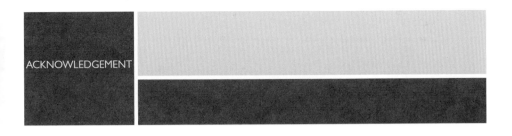

ACKNOWLEDGEMENT

This work began with an idea of producing an easy-to-use revision aid for the new MRCPsych exams. The compilation, drafting and research work behind the production of these MCQs were inspired by a number of colleagues and friends. We are thankful to all of them and we hope we will be able to deliver what they envisaged throughout the making of this book.

Prof Rajarathinam inspired LP to take up psychiatry—not only as a profession to practice, but an experience to cherish and impart. If this book helps at least one motivated trainee to sustain his interest and take him closer to practicing psychiatry as a profession lifelong, we will rejoice that Prof. Rajarathinam's effort has not been wasted.

Dr Thambirajah helped us throughout the production of this book. Dr Kopal Tandon reviewed the genetics chapter and we are grateful for her thoughtful comments. Dr Niruj Ahuja from Newcastle helped us to ensure delivery of accurate facts based on high quality of evidence while preparing the chapter on epidemiology. Numerous trainees from Newcastle, Derby, and Nottingham helped us to constantly revise the content through their first hand experience of the exam. A special thanks to Dr Albert Michael for writing the foreword.

Heartfelt thanks to Priya and Sindhu. Their patience with our late working nights and sacrifice of almost all 52 weekends of the last calendar year were phenomenal contributions to this book.

CONTENTS

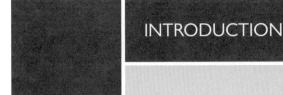

INTRODUCTION

MRCPsych exams are the most important exams a psychiatry trainee in the UK will sit during his or her career. Passing the MRCPsych is the most perceptible of the criteria that demonstrate the achievement of a number of competencies during the training.

WHO CAN SIT THE EXAM?

The details are clearly given in the Royal College website. They are summarized below for quick reference. Please note that these are subject to change and so we recommend checking with information at http://www.rcpsych.ac.uk before you apply.

Training requirements[1,2]
Candidates must have completed the mandatory training period of 12 months of post foundation training in psychiatry by the date of sitting the written exams. The recommended time frame for attempting Paper 2 is when the candidate is 18 to 24 months into his or her training. Posts must be part of a programme of training approved by PMETB or recognized by the Hospital or Trusts as having specific time, programme (journal clubs, grand rounds, teaching, supervision, etc.) and funds allocated for training. Individual posts can be of either 4 or 6 months' duration. In addition, the college also has placed emphasis on successful completion of the annual review of competency progression (ARCP) and other work place based assessments (WPBA) to be eligible for training. *The exact details need be confirmed from the college website as they are subject to regular reviews.*

WHAT IS PAPER 2?

The MRCPsych Paper 2 is 3 hours long and contains 200 questions. The paper consists of multiple choice questions (MCQ = 75%) and extended matching items (EMI = 25%). MCQs are in the 'best of five' (BOF) format. A best of five MCQ comprises a question stem of varying length, followed by a list of five options. Candidates should choose the single best option that answers the question.

The college has retained the EMI format from the previous pattern in the new format. An EMI comprises a specific theme (sometimes with a short description), followed by a set of answer choices (often in an alphabetical order) and a lead-in statement explaining what the candidate is being asked to do. This lead-in statement is then followed by a question list, set out in a logical order. The questions may be asked in form of clinical vignettes. The candidate may be required to choose more than one answer from the list of options for an individual question; in this case, the number of correct options will be clearly marked adjacent to the question.

Topics/syllabus for the Paper 2 exam
Neurosciences
  Neuroanatomy
  Neuropathology
  Neurophysiology

Neuroendocrinology
Neurochemistry
Neuroimaging
Developmental neuroscience

Psychopharmacology
Pharmacokinetics
Pharmacodynamics
Adverse reactions
Theories of action
Drug dependence
New drugs
Pharmacogenetics

Genetics
Cellular genetics
Molecular genetics
Behavioural genetics
Endophenotypes
Genetic epidemiology
Gene–environment interaction

Epidemiology
Surveys across the lifespan
Measures

Advanced psychological processes and treatments
Neuropsychology
Personality and personality disorder
Developmental psychopathology (including temperament)
Therapy models, methods, processes and outcomes
(BT, CBT, Family/couples, Interpersonal, Psychoanalytic, Psychoeducation)
Treatment adherence
Psychosocial influences

HOW TO PREPARE FOR THE EXAM

The MRCPsych journey starts the very day the training starts. This should be directed towards gaining the requirements towards sitting the exam, as well as getting a good knowledge of the theories that underlie the principles and practice of psychiatry. Reading for MRCPsych Paper 2 should ideally start as soon as one passes MRCPsych Paper 1. It is best to start reading around the cases that a trainee sees on a daily basis at the out-patient clinics and in-patient unit. These cases could be discussed with the supervisor and used for case-based discussions. A good place would be to start with epidemiology. For example, one could discuss risk factors for a particular clinical condition seen in a patient during a supervision session. In the process, the trainee can read around incidence and prevalence rates from standard sources such as the *British Journal of Psychiatry*. This process will help cultivate a regular journal-reading habit. So by 6 to 8 months after passing Paper 1, a trainee could familiarize him or herself with most of epidemiology, neurosciences, advanced psychology, genetics, and advanced psychopharmacology, which are covered in Paper 2. It will be a good idea to get the timetable and the topics at the local deanery MRCPsych course and read the relevant material before going in for the teaching sessions. This is particularly relevant for psychology (where we may not get a lot of opportunity to discuss topics with a psychologist in clinical practice) and neurosciences. In our experience, often the topics covered at teaching sessions do not correlate with exam syllabi or exam schedules. This can be particularly difficult and has to be taken into consideration during the study period.

Some of the most challenging topics for the Paper 2 exam include neurosciences, epidemiology, and genetics. In our opinion, one must leave no stone unturned when preparing for these topics. These topics are especially challenging as one does not deal with them routinely in the everyday practice of psychiatry. A substantial period must be devoted to prepare for these topics.

During the final 8–10 weeks preceding the exam, it would be best to create a timetable, with the syllabus and curriculum in mind, so as not to leave out important topics. Reading during this period should be exam-oriented and should be done along with practice multiple choice questions. This could be done on your own or in a study group. Preparing in a group helps to get an idea of where one stands with respect to the knowledge base.

Practice tests

A number of revision courses are now available for the new MRCPsych exams. Revision courses and materials could be used only to aid rapid revision and synthesize exam techniques. But it is best to revise from material the candidate has already read during the previous 10 months, rather than starting afresh. The MRCPsych exam prepares a psychiatric trainee for lifelong learning. It is best not to rely exclusively on 1 or 2 days of cramming to gain knowledge that sets your career on track.

It is very beneficial to take a number of mock and practice tests before the exam as these will give a fairly good idea of one's strengths and weaknesses. Look out for mock exams conducted by industry sponsors and local tutors. If possible, request your senior colleagues to organize a mock exam. It is best to do mock exams under the actual exam conditions, that is in paper and pencil format, using 200 questions and timing it at 180 minutes.

Books to read

Knowledge is not derived from textbooks alone. All kinds of resources are useful, including the internet, but it is best to base the core reading on standard textbooks. These textbooks should form the basis of reading, but reading should not be restricted to these.

The two reference books that we recommend are *Kaplan and Sadock's Comprehensive Textbook of Psychiatry* (this is an American book, which is comprehensive, with DSM and ICD criteria, and forms excellent reading in psychology, psychopharmacology, and neurosciences in addition to clinical psychiatry) and the *New Oxford Textbook of Psychiatry* (the latest edition is on its way). Both are two-volume textbooks and are useful for all parts of the exams. For core text revision, the *Shorter Oxford Textbook of Psychiatry* is a very good book. Each chapter is written in an authoritative style and is relevant to training in the UK. At the end of each section or topic there is a reference for further reading on the topic, which is invaluable. Most psychiatric epidemiology is covered extensively in these textbooks.

A good introductory textbook for psychopharmacology is Stephen Stahl's *Essential Psychopharmacology: Neuroscientific Basis and Practical Applications*. It is very lucid to read with a number of diagrams, which help understanding of the basis of psychopharmacology.

There are a number of books for basic psychology. *Psychology: Themes and Variations* by Wayne Weiten is especially recommended. It is an American book which is very easy to read with a lot of examples. Thambirajah's *Psychological Basis of Psychiatry* is also a good book, specifically designed for MRCPsych exams. These books should be of use for both Papers 1 and 2. In addition, these reference books give a good account of psychological tests and psychotherapies.

Basic neuroscience is a difficult subject to revise; most of us lose touch with the volatile facts regarding anatomy and physiology of the central nervous system. A good bet would be to use the same books that you used for undergraduate study for topics such as neurophysiology or neuroanatomy. Another fantastic resource, and especially recommended by the authors for all aspects of basic and clinical sciences, is the series of reviews produced by the American College of Neuropsychopharmacology under the title *Neuropsychopharmacology: the Fifth Generation of Progress*.

It is available, free of cost, online from the American College of Neuropsychopharmacology (ACNP) website. (Go to http://www.acnp.org and follow the link to publications.) This is also a good resource for basic genetics. Unfortunately, access for further updates of this resource now needs a paid subscription.

Genetics can be revised from reading the free-to-download book *Seminars in Psychiatric Genetics*, published by the Royal College. Please be aware that though it provides a good grounding for basic genetic concepts, it is nearly 16 years old and psychiatric genetics has moved well ahead of this book. An updated (2004) edition of *Psychiatric Genetics and Genomics*, edited by McGuffin *et al.* and published by Oxford University Press, is the best available resource for revising genetics for MRCPsych Paper 2 currently. For newer data, one must regularly skim through *Archives of General Psychiatry* and other such journals.

MRCPsych exam Paper 2 revision techniques in summary
1. Always stick to the standard textbooks you have read earlier. But remember textbooks are not written with the aim of helping trainees pass MRCPsych exams. So avoid spending too much time on irrelevant details.
2. As there is no bank of questions from previous papers for candidates to revise and attempt the exam confidently, one should get the basic concepts straight and correct, in order to tackle any surprises!
3. Group study helps in many ways; but make sure your peers are motivated to fully participate in the group.
4. Plan, plan, and plan! Structure your time according to the syllabus you have to revise. Spend equal time updating your knowledge from journals and solving MCQs.
5. There is no harm in utilizing all available materials before you attempt your exam—ask your senior ST trainees or colleagues and seek resources from revision courses and local MRCPsych teaching lectures.

APPROACH TO MULTIPLE CHOICE QUESTIONS[3,4]

The MRCPsych exam is more than reading and understanding the core subject. It has also to do with the technique of attempting best- of- five MCQs. Unlike the old-style ISQ, the new style is a bit more difficult to do because the chance of getting the answer wrong is 80% compared to 50% with the older style. The very concept of selecting the best answer lies in the fact that there may be more than one right answer, but we need to choose the best answer. In order to do this, you get 180 minutes to answer 200 questions, that is less than 1 minute to answer a question. This means that the more familiar you are with the concepts, the faster you can answer and you will be able to spend more time on the more difficult and longer questions. It is said that in most medical examinations, candidates who answer half the questions correctly would score around the 50th or 60th percentile. A score of 65% (130/200) would place the examinee above the 80th percentile, whereas a score of 30% (60/200) would rank him or her below the 15th percentile. Test performance will always be influenced by your test- taking skills. Considering various test- taking strategies, and developing and perfecting them well in advance of the test date can help you concentrate better on the test itself. We recommend you try various techniques to find what works best for you. It should, in the end, help you to:
• increase your reading pace;
• focus on the most relevant information;
• eliminate as many options as possible when you are not sure of the correct answer.
You require enough practice using the techniques so that it becomes second nature and you don't concentrate on anything but how to choose the correct answer when you actually sit the exam.

Timing

Time management is an important skill for exam success. As mentioned above, the test has 200 questions to be answered in 3 hours, which leaves about 54 seconds per question. Each time you spend more than 54 seconds on a single question, time should be made up on other questions. Therefore it is essential to practise answering questions within a time limit to avoid pacing errors in the exam. This is where attempting a number of mock exams will help.

Approaching each question

There are several established techniques for tackling multiple choice questions which will help you in finding the single best answer choice. One of these is classifying each question as easy, workable, or impossible. The basic aim in doing this is to

• answer all easy questions;
• figure out the answer to all the workable questions in a reasonable amount of time;
• make fast and intelligent guesses on the impossible ones.

Another technique is to read the answer choices first along with the last sentence of the question before reading through the question quickly, so as to extract the most relevant information as well as to consider each of the answer possibilities in the context of the question. This is especially relevant when the question stem is large, for example a case scenario.

Elimination is one of the best tools that can be used in a single best answer multiple choice exam. Excluding the possibility of one answer choice proportionately increases the probability of choosing the right answer.

Since this is a paper and pencil exam, it is better to answer the questions in order, one by one; this reduces the chance of skipping and accidentally marking the wrong question or skipping an item. To avoid these 'frame-shift' errors, answer difficult questions with your best guess, mark them for review, move on and come back to them if you have time at the end.

Random guessing

• There are no negative marks for wrong answers, so no question should be left unanswered.
• A hunch is probably better than a random guess; we also suggest selecting a choice which you recognize over another which is totally unfamiliar to you.
• It is never beneficial to pick random choices unless you are grossly out of time and not answering all the questions, in which case the best bet would be to select a single letter like 'C' and marking the remaining questions with it. It is obvious that in this case the chance of picking the correct answer decreases with more answer choices. It is also believed that MCQ makers prefer to hide the answers either in C or D, the middle-most choices, more often than in the periphery. (However, it should be noted that the college is trying to get rid of this bias by presenting the multiple choices in alphabetical order.)
• It is also very important to not randomly guess the answers during your study and review sessions as well as the practice test sessions, as it may increase the tendency to do the same for the exam.
• As mentioned before, it is essential to take as many practice tests as possible to try the various techniques and select the ones that give you the best results.
• Use any extra time you might have to recheck your answers. Do not be casual in your review or you may overlook serious mistakes.
• Never give up. If you begin to feel frustrated try taking a 30-second breather. Remember your goals and keep in mind the effort and time you have spent in preparing for the exam compared with the small additional effort you will need to keep your focus and concentration throughout the exam.

Other things to do before the exam

Make arrangements for study leaves as early as possible. It is also important to find out how much private study leave you are entitled to. Make all the necessary swaps on the on call rota. Some deaneries arrange for stay and transport for the exam if there are a number of candidates taking the exam. Application forms should be sent well in time. If there are queries regarding applications, they should be clarified with the college at the earliest.

The day prior to exam, choose a good place to stay near the centre, even if it is expensive. As usual, it is important to get a good night's sleep. A good preparation should make you feel confident.

BOF MCQ exam techniques in summary

1. People who fail in MCQ exams do so not because they don't know the answer for some questions; it is because they think they know the answer and keep thinking about one question for 5 minutes or so, losing the remaining time to answer the rest.
2. All questions carry one mark only, no matter how easy or difficult each one is. So why spend all your time on 'difficult' ones?
3. In large, clinical vignette type of questions you may have many irrelevant details; at the same time you may also have valuable clues to solve the BOF. It is useful to read the last sentence of the question quickly, before reading the large vignettes fully.
4. People have different styles of approaching BOF. Exclusion technique needs more time than direct answer picking; if your style is one of exclusion, make sure you practise well enough to carry this out faster during the exam.

AFTER THE EXAM

If you have some stamina left at the end of this huge ordeal, it is not a bad idea to start recollecting the questions to form a question bank which will be useful for future candidates. It is best to recollect the questions in the company of a couple of colleagues. It will be a good idea to get the questions back to the college tutor and this will help to arrange further teaching. This will also help you to prepare for Paper 3 in the future.

READING LIST

Reference books and core clinical psychiatry

Gelder MG et al., eds. Shorter Oxford Textbook of Psychiatry, 5th edn. Oxford University Press, 2006.
Gelder MG et al., eds. New Oxford Textbook of Psychiatry, 2nd edn. Oxford University Press, 2009.
Sadock BJ and Sadock VA. Kaplan and Sadock's Synopsis of Psychiatry: Behavioral Sciences/Clinical Psychiatry, 10th edn. Lippincott Williams and Wilkins, 2007.
Kaplan HA, Sadock BJ, and Sadock VA, eds. Kaplan and Sadock's Comprehensive Textbook of Psychiatry, Vols 1 and 2. Lippincott Williams and Wilkins, 2004.

Neurosciences, psychopharmacology, and genetics

Stahl SM. Essential Psychopharmacology: Neuroscientific Basis and Practical Application, 3rd edn. Cambridge University Press, 2008.
Taylor D, Paton C, and Kerwin R. The Maudsley Prescribing Guidelines . Informa Healthcare, 2007.
Davis K, Charney D, et al. ACNP Neuropsychopharmacology—the fifth generation of progress (free resource online at http://www.acnp.com).
McGuffin P, Owen MJ, and Gottesman II, eds. Psychiatric Genetics and Genomics. Oxford University Press, 2004.
Cummings JL and Mega MS, eds. Neuropsychiatry and Behavioural Neuroscience. Oxford University Press, 2003.

Advanced psychology

Weiten W. *Psychology: Themes and Variations*, 3rd edn. Brooks/Cole, 1995.

Thambirajah MS. *Psychological Basis of Psychiatry*. Elsevier, 2005.

[1] http://rcpsych.ac.uk/PDF/Exams%20Eligibility%20July%202008.pdf
[2] http://rcpsych.ac.uk/exams/about/mrcpsychpaperii.aspx
[3] Bhushan V and Le T. *First Aid for the USMLE Step 1*, 16th edn. McGraw Hill Higher Education, 2006.
[4] Stein M and Hwang G. *Cracking the Boards: USMLE Step 1*, 3rd edn. Princeton Review Series, 2000.

1. It has been demonstrated that the levels of monoamine metabolites in CSF varies with polymorphism of serotonin transporter protein. Which of the following components of genetic apparatus is responsible for such polymorphisms?

   A. Non-coding sequences
   B. RNA
   C. Exons
   D. Ribosomes
   E. Chromosomal count

2. In the diagnosis of HIV, following a positive ELISA test, western blotting could be used to confirm the diagnosis. Which of the following cellular components is separated by electrophoresis for western blotting?

   A. Proteins
   B. RNA
   C. DNA
   D. Cell membrane lipids
   E. Free amino acids

3. Genetic information in an organism is inherited equally from parents of both sexes. An exception to this is seen in

   A. Ribosomal RNA
   B. Small arms of chromosomes
   C. Mitochondrial DNA
   D. Coding sequences of nuclear DNA
   E. Non-coding sequences of nuclear DNA

4. Microtubule-associated protein tau undergoes several post-translational modifications and aggregates into paired helical filaments in Alzheimer's disease. These modifications of tau include all of the following except

   A. Hyperphosphorylation
   B. Protein glycosylation
   C. Ubiquitination
   D. Polyamination
   E. Amino acid activation

5. **Which one of the following refers to the synthesis of RNA molecules from DNA?**

   A. Replication
   B. Translation
   C. Transcription
   D. Splicing
   E. Modification

6. **Newly synthesized RNA molecules undergo splicing to produce mRNA. Which one of the following best describes the process of splicing?**

   A. Introns are removed, exons are joined together.
   B. Introns and exons are randomly spliced and pasted.
   C. Both introns and exons are spliced out to make the RNA compact.
   D. Splicing takes place in cytoplasm.
   E. Splicing is a reversible process.

7. **Which one of the following stages of the cell cycle is dominant in non-dividing cells such as neurones?**

   A. Synthetic phase (S)
   B. Gap phase 1 (G1)
   C. Gap phase 0 (G0)
   D. Gap phase 2 (G2)
   E. Mitotic phase (M)

8. **Which one of the following nitrogenous bases is present in RNA but not DNA?**

   A. Adenine
   B. Guanine
   C. Cytosine
   D. Thymidine
   E. Uracil

9. **Gene cloning is the process of insertion of foreign DNA into a replicating sequence such as a plasmid. Which of the following is essential for successful cloning?**

   A. Restriction enzyme
   B. Actively meiotic cell
   C. RNA ligase
   D. Stem cell
   E. Ovum

10. **Polymerase chain reaction (PCR) was used in a study to search for various viruses in hippocampal tissue and CSF of patients with schizophrenia. PCR is the preferred method for the above study due to which of the following properties?**

    A. A small sample of DNA is sufficient to be detected by PCR.
    B. PCR is useful even if viral sequences are not known previously.
    C. PCR is not altered by contamination from other viruses in the lab.
    D. Each amplification procedure using PCR can be completed within a few months.
    E. The DNA replication process using PCR is relatively error free.

11. **In a child with flat occiput, Brushfield spots, and simian palmar creases, the most common cause of death is**

    A. Cardiac failure
    B. Leukaemia
    C. Hypothyroidism
    D. Suicide
    E. Accidental injury

12. **A child with low-set ears, polydactyly, and coloboma of the iris is diagnosed to have Patau's syndrome. Which of the following chromosomal aberrations explains this presentation?**

    A. Meiotic non-disjunction
    B. Mitotic non-disjunction
    C. Reduplication of chromosome 13
    D. Amplification of the long arm of chromosome 18
    E. Partial deletion of chromosome 18

13. **Heritability is often used to express the genetic contribution in a multifactorial disease. Which of the following best describes heritability?**

    A. It refers to the share of genes contributing to a phenotype in an individual patient.
    B. Heritability is disease specific and is always a fixed measure for a population.
    C. Zero heritability excludes the possibility of finding a genetic locus underlying causation.
    D. Identification of a genetic locus is necessary to estimate heritability.
    E. Heritability cannot be measured for polygenic disorders.

14. **The risk of severe affective disorder in relatives of probands with bipolar affective disorder is**

    A. 40%
    B. 55%
    C. 78%
    D. 19%
    E. 5%

15. **Which of the following chromosomal abnormalities results in a phenotype with a cat-like cry and facial dysmorphism?**
    A. Partial deletion chromosome 5
    B. Partial deletion chromosome 15
    C. Trisomy chromosome 5
    D. Trisomy chromosome 15
    E. Non-disjunction chromosome 1

16. **Which of the following polymorphism has been linked to performance on working memory tasks in patients with schizophrenia?**
    A. MAO-A polymorphism
    B. COMT polymorphism
    C. 5-HT transporter promoter region
    D. Apolipoprotein E polymorphism
    E. MAO-B polymorphism

17. **Which one of the following processes can inactivate a gene?**
    A. Methylation
    B. Crossing over
    C. Uncoiling of a chromosome
    D. Unwinding of DNA strands
    E. Condensation

18. **Expression of genes depending upon the parent of origin is a phenomenon seen in**
    A. Genomic imprinting
    B. Genetic anticipation
    C. Genetic amplification
    D. Autosomal aneuploidy
    E. Fragmented penetrance

19. **Which of the following clinical scenarios is most likely to be a result of genetic anticipation?**
    A. Advanced maternal age increases the risk of Down's syndrome.
    B. Mitochondrial disorders are transmitted only from mothers.
    C. Successive generations display the phenotype of Huntington's chorea at an earlier age.
    D. An autosomal recessive disorder presents with a mild dysfunction in heterozygous individuals.
    E. Male fetuses with one copy of a mutant X chromosome often die *in utero*.

20. **A large pedigree is observed for the occurrence of a rare form of recurrent strokes. All affected females in the pedigree produce affected children of both sexes. But none of the affected males pass the disease on to the next generation. The most likely mode of inheritance is**
    A. X-linked dominant
    B. X-linked recessive
    C. Mitochondrial
    D. Autosomal recessive
    E. Spontaneous mutations

21. **Which of the following conditions will produce more than one Barr body in cells of affected patients?**
    A. Testicular feminization syndrome
    B. Sexual infantilism due to Turner's syndrome
    C. Bilateral gynaecomastia due to Kleinfelter's syndrome (47 XXY)
    D. Triple-X syndrome with normal fertility
    E. Fragile-X syndrome

22. **Mrs Smith is a 32-year-old woman with normal IQ scores whose son has been recently diagnosed to have fragile-X syndrome. There is no family history of fragile-X syndrome in her husband's lineage, but Mrs Smith's maternal uncle had mental retardation, suspected to be fragile X retrospectively. Which of the following best describes Mrs Smith's genotype?**
    A. She has a premutation.
    B. She has a complete mutation which is unexpressed.
    C. She is completely normal in terms of her genotype.
    D. She does not have a mutation due to variable penetrance of fragile-X syndrome.
    E. She has a fragile-X chromosome whose expression will occur only after age 40.

23. **If a mother has alleles 'pp' while a father has alleles 'Pp' at the same locus, then which of the following distributions can be expected in the next generation?**
    A. 1/2 Pp, 1/2 pp
    B. 1/3 Pp, 2/3 pp
    C. 1/2 PP, 1/2 pp
    D. 1/2 Pp, 1/2 PP
    E. 1/4 Pp, 3/4 pp

24. Which of the following genetic abnormalities is associated with rocker bottom feet, protrusion of bowel through the umbilical cord, and low-set ears in a male child, newly born to both healthy parents with no history of genetic disorders in the family?

    A. Deletion
    B. Insertion
    C. Nonsense mutation
    D. Translocation
    E. Aneuploidy

25. Which of the following genetic mechanisms can explain the occurrence of Angelman's syndrome?

    A. Maternal disomy of chromosome 15
    B. Paternal disomy of chromosome 15
    C. Spontaneous deletion of one copy of an allele at a certain locus, derived from the father
    D. Spontaneous deletion of both copies of alleles from the father and mother
    E. All of the above

26. If p is the frequency of allele A and q is the frequency of allele B of the same gene, then the frequency of the heterozygous combination AB is

    A. p^2
    B. q^2
    C. pq
    D. 2pq
    E. 4pq

27. The criteria for defining a trait as endophenotype include all of the following except

    A. Association with a candidate gene.
    B. Cosegregation with increased relative risk of the trait in relatives.
    C. The expression is dependent on the clinical state of the patient.
    D. The endophenotype is more common in the patient's relatives than the general population.
    E. The trait and disease have a biologically plausible association.

28. The fusion of two different chromosomes at a common centromere results from which of the following?

    A. Robertsonian translocation
    B. Reciprocal translocation
    C. Inversion
    D. Duplication
    E. Iso-chromosome formation

29. **Which of the following best describes multifactorial diseases?**
    A. Diseases caused by multiple environmental factors
    B. Diseases caused by multiple genetic factors
    C. Disease caused by non-genetic, non-environmental causes
    D. Diseases caused by the interaction of multiple genes and environmental factors
    E. None of the above

30. **A husband and wife are both affected by an autosomal dominant disorder with 75% penetrance. Provided that they are both heterozygous for the mutation, what will be the influence of this less than 100% penetrance rate on the likelihood that their children will be affected?**
    A. Likelihood of having unaffected offspring remains unchanged
    B. Likelihood of having unaffected offspring increases
    C. Likelihood of having unaffected offspring decreases
    D. Likelihood of having unaffected offspring depends on the sex of the offspring
    E. Likelihood of having unaffected offspring depends on the birth order of the offspring

31. **Which one of the following statement is false with respect to Mendelian inheritance?**
    A. The law of independent assortment is a Mendelian principle.
    B. Segregation of genetic traits is explained by Mendelian principles.
    C. Mendelian principles are based on continuous variables.
    D. Mendelian principles are applicable to human genetics.
    E. The law of uniformity is a Mendelian principle.

32. **Which of the following patterns of inheritance can skip generations and can affect individuals with unaffected parents?**
    A. Autosomal dominant with complete penetrance
    B. Autosomal recessive
    C. X-linked dominant
    D. Mitochondrial inheritance
    E. None of the above

33. **Which one of the following best describes a substitution mutation?**
    A. It is a frame-shift mutation.
    B. It is a point mutation.
    C. It results in the replacement of a random sequence of bases.
    D. It is often a nonsense mutation.
    E. Substitution occurs only in coding regions of DNA.

34. Fragile sites present in human chromosomes are demonstrated using deprivation of which one of the following components used in DNA synthesis?

    A. Thymidine
    B. Uric acid
    C. Thiamine
    D. Iron
    E. Magnesium

35. Which of the following is not an established candidate endophenotype for schizophrenia?

    A. Prepulse inhibition
    B. P50 suppression
    C. Corrective eye saccades
    D. Working memory capacity
    E. Duration of untreated psychosis

36. The existence of two or more different chromosomal sites where mutations result in the same clinical expression is called

    A. Allelic heterogeneity
    B. Locus heterogeneity
    C. Pleiotropy
    D. Variable penetration
    E. Variable expression

37. Which of the following factors is often corrected for when ascertaining probands and unaffected relatives for family genetic studies?

    A. Age of onset of the illness
    B. Severity of the illness
    C. Duration of the illness
    D. Birth order of affected probands
    E. All of the above

38. A researcher studying the genetic explanation for delusional disorder detects genes at two different loci in the sample studied. One gene modifies the expression of the other in producing the delusional disorder phenotype. This phenomenon is called

    A. Epistasis
    B. Variable expression
    C. Incomplete penetrance
    D. Haplotype expression
    E. Codominance

39. **The population distribution curve of a multifactorial trait is such that when it crosses a threshold disease becomes manifest. A similar distribution curve for relatives of affected individuals will be**

   A. Shifted to the right
   B. Narrower in size
   C. Broader in size
   D. Shifted to the left
   E. Taller peak

40. **In spite of accumulating evidence for the role played by genetic factors in various psychiatric illnesses, this is not translated to clinical genetic approaches in psychiatry. This paucity is most probably related to**

   A. The magnitude of gene–illness association has an odds ratios around 20 to 50 for most psychiatric disorders.
   B. Associations between genes and phenotypes are less specific in psychiatry.
   C. Gene–disorder association is not contingent on environment in psychiatry.
   D. The causal chain from genes to psychiatric disorders is too short to be explored in detail.
   E. All of the above.

41. **A 40-year-old Caucasian lady presents with depression. Which one of the following genotypes will be associated with better treatment response to SSRIs?**

   A. Long/ long polymorphism in promoter region of the serotonin transporter gene
   B. Short/ short polymorphism in the coding region of the serotonin transporter gene
   C. Long/ long polymorphism in the coding region of the serotonin transporter gene
   D. Long/ long polymorphism in the coding region of the 5-HT$_{2A}$ receptor
   E. None of the above

42. **A child suffers from moderate learning disability, facial rash, and renal and lung cysts. He has coffee-coloured patches on his skin with intractable seizures. The mode of inheritance of this disease is**

   A. X-linked dominant
   B. X-linked recessive
   C. Autosomal dominant
   D. Autosomal recessive
   E. Chromosomal translocation

43. **A 21-year-old man with mental retardation and features of autism, enlarged external ears, and protruding jaw is most likely to show which of the following genetic abnormalities?**

   A. CGG repeats
   B. CAG repeats
   C. XY repeats
   D. GAG repeats
   E. AAT repeats

44. **The existence of two or more different mutant alleles at the same locus, resulting in varied clinical expression is called**
    A. Allelic heterogeneity
    B. Locus heterogeneity
    C. Pleiotropy
    D. Variable penetration
    E. Variable expression

45. **Which of the following describes the phenomenon that the same gene has two or more different effects?**
    A. Allelic heterogeneity
    B. Locus heterogeneity
    C. Pleiotropy
    D. Variable penetration
    E. Variable expression

46. **A mutation where insertion or deletion of a base pair results in mistranslation of the genetic code beyond that point is called a**
    A. Frame-shift mutation
    B. Silent mutation
    C. Nonsense mutation
    D. In-frame mutation
    E. Point mutation

47. **Which of the following genetic analyses studies the departure from independent segregation?**
    A. Restriction fragment length polymorphism
    B. Linkage analysis
    C. Adoption studies
    D. Fluorescent *in situ* hybridization
    E. Twin studies

48. **In genetic linkage studies, the LOD score above which linkage is conventionally thought to be significant is**
    A. 10
    B. 5
    C. 100
    D. 3
    E. 2

49. In linkage analysis, LOD scores are used. Which of the following best describes the LOD score?

    A. It is the log of the ratio of the likelihood of a specific recombination fraction to the likelihood that the recombination fraction is 1.
    B. It is the log of the ratio of the likelihood of the recombination fraction being 1 to the likelihood of a different specific recombination fraction.
    C. It is the log of the ratio of the likelihood of a specific recombination fraction to the likelihood that the recombination fraction is 1/2.
    D. It is the log of the ratio of the likelihood of a specific recombination fraction to the likelihood that the recombination fraction is zero.
    E. It is the log of the ratio of the likelihood of a specific recombination fraction to the likelihood that the recombination fraction is log of 1.

50. Two possible alleles of a gene are A and B. The genotype is distributed as AA, AB, and BB in the population. In a sample of 100 people, if the genotype frequency of AA is 40, AB is 54, and BB is 6, then the frequency of allele B is

    A. 60
    B. 12
    C. 66
    D. 33
    E. 120

51. A phenotypically indistinguishable disorder occurring in the absence of the genotype is called

    A. Phenocopy
    B. Pleiotropy
    C. Heterogeneity
    D. Genocopy
    E. None of the above

52. Considering the Hardy–Weinberg equation in population genetics, which of the following assumptions are made?

    A. No inbreeding in the population
    B. No migration in the population
    C. No mutation in the population
    D. No selection against a phenotype
    E. All of the above

53. **RNA is synthesized from DNA in most the normal circumstances. Which of the following enzymes catalyses the synthesis of DNA from RNA?**

    A. DNA ligase
    B. RNA polymerase
    C. Reverse transcriptase
    D. Primase
    E. DNA polymerase I

54. **Equatorial alignment of chromosomes takes place in which of the following stages of mitosis?**

    A. Prophase
    B. Anaphase
    C. Metaphase
    D. Telophase
    E. Interphase

55. **Condensation of chromatin material, resulting in the production of sister chromatids, takes place in**

    A. Prophase
    B. Anaphase
    C. Metaphase
    D. Telophase
    E. Interphase

56. **According to the Hardy–Weinberg law, if a population has 1 in 1600 of its members affected by a homozygous recessive disorder, how many members will be heterozygous carriers?**

    A. 1 in 40
    B. 39 in 40
    C. 1 in 80
    D. 1 in 20
    E. 1 in 4800

57. **Nucleic acids constitute the chemical base of genes. Which of the following is not a component of nucleic acids?**

    A. Pentose sugar
    B. Phosphate groups
    C. Purines
    D. Pyrimidines
    E. Arachidonic acid

58. **Which of the following genetic studies compares the frequency of a marker in groups of patients versus unrelated controls?**

A. Association study
B. Linkage study
C. Family study
D. Adoption study
E. Ecological study

59. **In genetic twin studies, pair-wise concordance differs from proband-wise concordance in that**

A. Pair-wise concordance calculates the total number of concordant affected pairs.
B. Pair-wise concordance calculates the total number of affected individual cotwins.
C. Proband-wise concordance can not be assessed in multifactorial disorders.
D. Proband-wise concordance is useful only in dizygotes.
E. All of the above.

60. **The ratio of clinically affected to unaffected offspring for an autosomal recessive disorder where both parents are carriers is**

A. 1 : 1
B. 1 : 3
C. 3 : 1
D. 2 : 1
E. 1 : 2

61. **Variation in the expected gene frequency in a population can be explained using all of the following except**

A. Gene drift
B. Gene flow
C. Natural selection
D. Spontaneous mutation
E. Increased death rate

62. **A study finds that monozygotic concordance of intelligence is 0.86 while dizygotic concordance is 0.61. The heritability of intelligence is given by**

A. 0.5
B. 0.25
C. 0.025
D. 0.07
E. 1.131

63. **All of the following show non-Mendelian inheritance except**
    A. Leber's optic neuropathy
    B. Huntington's disease
    C. Angelman's syndrome
    D. Prader–Willi syndrome
    E. Cystic fibrosis

64. **Which one of the following methods is used in the determination of environment versus genetic contribution to a phenotype?**
    A. Angoff method
    B. Receiver operator curve
    C. Path analysis
    D. Bonferroni method
    E. Diffusion method

65. **The proportion of the total phenotypic variance accounted for by additive gene effects is called**
    A. Broad heritability
    B. Narrow heritability
    C. Concordance
    D. Genetic determination
    E. Gene–environment covariance

66. **Mutations on chromosome 17 are linked to which of the following neurodegenerative disorders?**
    A. Huntington's disease
    B. Lewy body dementia
    C. Frontotemporal dementia
    D. Alzheimer's dementia
    E. Crutzfeld–Jakob disease

67. **A 24-year-old man suffers from repeated episodes of sleepiness associated with sudden falls. Which of the following polymorphisms is associated with this patient's condition?**
    A. Dopamine D2 receptor polymorphism
    B. CYP2D6 polymorphism
    C. CYP3A4 polymorphism
    D. HLA DR2 polymorphism
    E. Serotonin transporter polymorphism

68. **Which of the following genotypes has been shown to influence antisocial outcomes in maltreated children?**
    A. Low COMT activity
    B. High MAO-B activity
    C. 5-HT transporter long variant
    D. High MAO-A activity
    E. DRD3 Ser9Gly polymorphism

69. **Which of the following features predicts a good response to lithium treatment in bipolar patients with acute mania?**
    A. Dysphoric mania
    B. Mixed episode of mania and depression
    C. Mania during a rapid cycling phase
    D. Classical mania without schizoaffective features
    E. Family history of bipolar disorder

70. **A 13-year-old boy presents with slow and clumsy walking and difficulties in writing. On examination he has a slurred speech with high stepping and a wide-based gait. Deep tendon reflexes are absent and plantar responses are extensor bilaterally. Which of the following chromosomes is implicated in the aetiology?**
    A. Chromosome 1
    B. Chromosome 14
    C. Chromosome 4
    D. Chromosome 7
    E. Chromosome 9

71. **Family aggregation is an important source of evidence for psychiatric genetics. Which of the following is true with regard to genetic relatedness?**
    A. A 25% decrement in risk across successive generations suggests an environmental contribution for the disease studied.
    B. First degree relatives share 75% of their genes.
    C. In multifactorial diseases >50% decrement in risk across successive generations is seen.
    D. The expression λ (lambda) refers to linkage disequilibrium.
    E. Second-degree relatives share 50% of their genes.

72. **The proportion of phenotypic variation attributable to non-genetic causes among depressed patients is**
    A. 30–40%
    B. 40–50%
    C. 90–95%
    D. 60–65%
    E. 10–20%

73. **Which of the following is true regarding the** *APOE* **gene in Alzheimer's disease?**
    A. *APOE ε4* increases the risk of Alzheimer's disease in a dose-dependent fashion.
    B. *APOE ε4* confers a protective effect against vascular dementia.
    C. *APOE ε3* variant offers a protective effect against Alzheimer's dementia.
    D. The odds of Alzheimer's disease in subjects with one copy of *APOE ε4* is 15 times higher.
    E. The frequency of *APOE ε4* in the general population is extremely rare.

74. **Which of the following genes implicated in schizophrenia potentially modulates D-amino acid oxidase?**
    A. *NRG1*
    B. *BDNF*
    C. *G72*
    D. *DISC1*
    E. *DMD* (Dystrophin)

75. **A transcriptome refers to**
    A. All DNA in a cell
    B. All expressed mRNA in a cell
    C. All expressed tRNA in a cell
    D. All histones in a cell
    E. All introns in a cell

76. **Which of the following statements comparing the genetics of simple Mendelian disorders and schizophrenia is true?**
    A. Schizophrenia has higher monozygotic concordance.
    B. Phenocopies are probably more common in schizophrenia than in Mendelian disorders.
    C. Locus heterogeneity within families is very common in Mendelian disorders.
    D. Penetrance is almost always complete in schizophrenia.
    E. Mendelian disorders always present in childhood.

77. **The term copy number variation refers to**
    A. Differences in the number of copies of certain genes per genome
    B. Differences in the total number of genes in a genome
    C. Differences in genetic code between two normal parents of a diseased child
    D. Variations in single nucleotides of a functional genetic code
    E. Variations in length of promoter regions of certain transcription factors

78. **From the following, chose the correct combination of trinucleotide repeats and fragile-X syndrome genotype.**
    A. 6 to 60 CGG repeats: premutation
    B. 61 to 200 CAG repeats: mutation
    C. 2 to 20 CGG repeats: permutation
    D. >200 CGG repeats: full mutation
    E. >49 CCG repeats: full mutation

79. **Which of the following statements regarding genetic testing for Huntington's disease is true?**
    A. Genetic testing cannot predict the probable age of onset of symptoms.
    B. Direct identification of the trinucleotide repeats is not possible using currently available genetic tests.
    C. Prenatal testing is not possible for a fetus of non-affected parents.
    D. The disease does not occur in those with no positive family history of Huntington's disease.
    E. Homozygotes are more severely affected than heterozygotes.

80. **A 12-year-old boy presents with clinical features consistent with hyperkinetic disorder with conduct problems. On examination, he has an abnormal spinal curvature. Psychometric testing reveals deficits in linguistic and visuospatial skills with borderline IQ. His younger brother has multiple, light-brown spots on his face. Which of the following is the likely mode of inheritance?**
    A. Autosomal dominant
    B. Autosomal recessive
    C. Trinucleotide expansion
    D. X-linked recessive
    E. X-linked dominant

1. A. Polymorphism refers to variations in the genome at a particular locus noted in a general, apparently healthy population. Polymorphisms occur at a fairly high frequency in the general population. When the polymorphism occurs in more than 1% of a population, it can be considered as useful for genetic linkage analysis. ABO blood groups are a good example of polymorphism expressed in the protein products of genes. Restriction fragment length polymorphisms are those variations that create or destroy the sites at which restriction enzymes act on a DNA molecule, rendering differences in the final 'restricted' or cleaved DNA when these enzymes are applied *in vitro*. If these polymorphisms are due to changes in a single nucleotide in a sequence, they are called SNPs or single nucleotide polymorphisms. SNPs seem to be one of the most common genetic variations and various SNP genotyping methods are being increasingly employed to study polymorphisms. Polymorphisms arise originally out of mutations but are maintained in populations due to factors such as founder effect, genetic drift, and natural selection. Note that most polymorphisms occur in non-coding regions (that is introns), as coding sequences (or exons) on mutation often produce disease phenotypes. Serotonin transporter polymorphisms have been identified in the promoter region, which is a non-coding part of DNA (5HTTLPR–5HT transporter linked promoter region). 5HTTLPR can be a short or long variant. In those with a short variant, the serotonin transporter expression is low; the short variant is speculated to be associated with a higher incidence of affective disorders, anxiety, and PTSD. But the evidence is inconclusive as most studies are case–control design with significant heterogeneity. In addition, structural brain changes in the form of gray matter volume reduction in areas important for emotional processing, such as the amygdala, have been noted in subjects with the short variant of the promoter region.

An altered number of chromosomes is termed aneuploidy.

Kato T. Molecular genetics of bipolar disorder and depression. *Psychiatry and Clinical Neurosciences* 2007; **61**: 3–19.
Sadock BJ and Sadock VA. *Kaplan and Sadock's Comprehensive Textbook of Psychiatry*, 8th edn. Lippincott Williams and Wilkins, 2005, p. 260.

2. A. Molecular analysis techniques include Southern, northern, and western blotting. Western blotting is used in protein analysis, for example to detect HIV antibodies. Northern blotting is used in RNA analysis, while Southern blotting is used in the analysis of DNA. Southern blotting was named after its founder, Professor Edwin Southern; the other names were given to differentiate among the various blotting techniques.

Hayes PC et al. Blotting techniques for the study of DNA, RNA, and proteins. *British Medical Journal* 1989; **299**: 965–968.

3. C.   Mitochondrial DNA is wholly inherited from the ovum. The sperm has no mitochondria in its 'head'; the 'head' is made of nuclear material and the acrosomal cap. The 'body' of sperm have many mitochondria which provide energy to propel the 'tail'. The 'body' and 'tail' are shed on entry of sperm into the ovum. Hence the mitochondria of an embryo are completely maternally derived. This is important in clinical genetics as mitochondrial DNA abnormalities result in various diseases, such as MELAS (mitochondrial myopathy, encephalopathy, lactic acidosis, and recurrent stroke syndrome) and Leber hereditary optic neuropathy. These diseases are purely maternally inherited. Mitochondrial DNA codes for 13 proteins involved in the respiratory chain in addition to 22 tRNAs and two ribosomal RNAs.

Leonard JV and Shapira AHV. Mitochondrial respiratory chain disorders I: mitochondrial DNA defects. *Lancet* 2000; **355**: 299–304.

4. E.   Amino acid activation is an important step in the translation of mRNA to proteins. As tRNAs enter the cytoplasm after release from the nucleus where they are synthesized, they are attached to specific amino acids according to the codon sequences. This is an energy-dependent process called amino acid activation. The energy stored in such activated amino acids is used in making peptide bonds during protein translation. Translation takes place in the cytoplasm on ribosomes, where specific mRNAs are involved. Translation includes three steps—initiation, elongation, and termination. The ribosome contains two sites—peptidyl P site where methionine-containing tRNA initially binds and aminoacyl A site where each new incoming tRNAs with activated amino acids can bind. In the elongation step amino acids are added one by one in a string-like fashion to produce proteins. Chain termination is signalled by one of three codons—UAA, UGA, or UAG. Following this protein synthesis (or sometimes simultaneously at one end of long proteins), post-translational modifications take place to transport the synthesized proteins to appropriate cellular sites. These modifications take place in endoplasmic reticulum and golgi bodies. This includes covalent modifications, protein folding, and tagging with signal peptides to dispatch to appropriate cellular destinations. Glycosylation, proteolysis, phosphorylation, gamma carboxylation, prenylation, ubiquitation, polyamination, and nitration are some of the recognized post-translational modifications. This process is essential in tagging wrongly folded or aberrant proteins to enter lysosomes for destruction.

Gong CX *et al.* Post-translational modifications of tau protein in Alzheimer's disease. *Journal of Neural Transmission* 2005; **112**: 813–838.

5. C.   Transcription refers to the synthesis of RNA from DNA. Translation refers to the production of proteins from RNA. Replication refers to the production of new DNA copies from template copies of DNA. Splicing refers to the removal of non-coding sequences of RNA following transcription. DNA contains both coding and non-coding sequences. To synthesize proteins, the code contained in exons (coding sequences) are required. The heterogeneous nuclear RNA, which contains both coding exons and non-coding introns, undergoes splicing by spliceosomes within the nucleus to produce mature mRNA. Modification refers to the post-translational changes in a protein molecule before it becomes functionally active.

McGuffin P *et al.*, eds. *Psychiatric Genetics and Genomics.* Oxford University Press, 2002, pp. 10–12.

6. A.   In splicing, the non-coding introns (intervening codons) are removed and exons are pasted together, producing a compact mRNA. This takes place in the nucleus. The splicing is carried out by small nuclear RNAs and protein complexes, which together constitute spliceosomes. This is an irreversible process as normally hnRNAs (heterogeneous nuclear RNAs) cannot be reassembled from mRNAs.

McGuffin P *et al.*, eds. *Psychiatric Genetics and Genomics.* Oxford University Press, 2002, p. 11.

7. C.   Each cell undergoes a natural cycle in terms of its replication and nucleic acid synthesis activity. The cell cycle consists of four separate phases: G1, S, G2, and M. G1 stands for growth phase 1, S for synthetic phase, G2 for growth phase 2 and M for mitosis phase. In mitosis the cellular material, including chromosomes, is divided between two daughter cells. Cells can leave G1 phase to enter a G0 phase, also called the quiescent phase as no replicatory activity takes place here. Most of these cells have temporarily or reversibly stopped dividing, for example liver parenchyma, in which case they enter G1 phase on stimulation. Cells such as neurones enter G0 phase indefinitely, but note that this dogma of absolute neuronal cell cycle dormancy is increasingly being challenged. A number of neurodegenerative diseases in humans, such as Pick's disease, intractable temporal lobe epilepsy, progressive supranuclear palsy, Lewy body disease, and Parkinson's disease, are thought to be associated with a few neurones retaining the ability to re-enter mitosis, thus disrupting the normal cell cycle.

Collins K, Jacks T, and Pavletich NP. The cell cycle and cancer. *Proceedings of the National Academy of Sciences* 1997; **94**: 2776–2778.

Zhu X, Raina AK, and Smith MA. Cell cycle events in neurons: Proliferation or death? *American Journal of Pathology* 1999; **155**: 327–329.

8. E.   DNA and RNA are the most important nucleic acids in the cellular machinery. These nucleic acids are composed of many nucleotides. Nucleotides are phosphorylated versions of nucleosides. Each nucleoside consists of two components: a nitrogenous base and a pentose sugar. There are two types of nitrogenous bases that can constitute a nucleoside—purines and pyrimidines. Purines include adenine and guanine. Pyrimidines include cytosine, uracil, and thymine. Thymine is usually found only in DNA while uracil is specific to RNA. DNA is double stranded with hydrogen-bonded base pairs. In DNA adenine always bonds with thymine (two hydrogen bonds) while cytosine bonds with guanine (three hydrogen bonds). As a result of this specific pairing, the amount of total purines is always equal to the total pyrimidines in normal DNA (Chargaff's rule).

McGuffin P *et al.*, eds. *Psychiatric Genetics and Genomics*. Oxford University Press, 2002, p. 5.

9. A.   Cloning is the process of copying; cloning laboratory animals refers to making identical genetic copies of the organisms while cloning a gene refers to producing identical copies of the gene. Gene cloning involves the insertion of foreign DNA into vectors such as bacterial plasmids or phages. Replication of these vectors then produces numerous identical copies of the cloned gene. In order to carry out successful cloning, a method of cutting DNA at specific sites to obtain the necessary genetic element is crucial. This is possible using restriction enzymes. DNA ligase (not RNA ligase) is used to paste the cut genetic element with plasmid DNA. A stem cell or ovum is not necessary for gene cloning. Active mitosis is sufficient to carry out cloning, thus meiosis is not necessary for gene cloning.

Kumar PJ and Clark ML. *Clinical Medicine*, 6th edn. Elsevier, 2006, p. 169.

10.A. PCR stands for polymerase chain reaction. It is an amplification process wherein a small amount of DNA sample is amplified many times to provide a supply for diagnostic analyses. The polymerization requires heat-stable DNA polymerase, obtained from *Thermus aquaticus*. Just one copy of a DNA sequence is sufficient to undertake PCR (at least theoretically). As it is extremely sensitive, contamination from other DNA present in the lab. environment (from bacteria, viruses, and DNA of lab. personnel) presents significant difficulties. As PCR requires the hybridization of primers to known sequences at either side of the region of interest (i.e. flanking regions), completely unknown sequences cannot be polymerized. DNA cloning by PCR can be performed in a few hours, using relatively unsophisticated equipment. Typically, a PCR reaction consists of 30 cycles containing a denaturation, synthesis and reannealing step, with an individual cycle typically taking 3–5 min in an automated thermal cycler. This compares favourably with the time required for cell-based DNA cloning, which may take weeks. PCR is not error free. The DNA polymerases used for PCR usually have no error correction mechanisms such as exonuclease activity. So, if an error is made, initially it may get amplified uncorrected, but this is less of a problem now with the availability of high-fidelity DNA polymerases.

McGuffin P et al., eds. *Psychiatric Genetics and Genomics*. Oxford University Press, 2002, pp. 21–22.

11.A. The presence of low, flat occiput, Brushfield spots, and simian palmar creases indicates Down's syndrome. The most common cause of death in children with Down's syndrome is cardiac failure. Though hypothyroidism is a common accompaniment, this is rarely fatal. Suicide is not a major cause of death in this group. In adults with Down's syndrome, most of whom obtain surgical correction for major cardiac anomalies at a younger age, leukaemia becomes a major killer.

Hermon C et al. for the Collaborative Study Group of Genetic Disorders. Mortality and cancer incidence in persons with Down's syndrome, their parents and siblings. *Annals of Human Genetics* 2001; **65**: 167–176.

12.A. Patau syndrome results from aneuploidy of chromosome 13 where three copies are found. This is due to non-disjunction of chromosome 13 during meiosis, mostly in the mother. Similar to Down's, Patau's syndrome is associated with increasing maternal age. Patau's syndrome may also occur as a result of random non-disjunction during early cell division, resulting in a mosaic cell population. Rarely, Patau's syndrome can result from a translocation that leaves the fetus with three copies of chromosome 13. This is often a balanced translocation where almost no significant clinical changes are seen in the carrier, but this can affect the children of the carrier. In non-translocation-related Patau's syndrome, the chances of a couple having another child with trisomy 13 is less than 1%. Most fetuses with trisomy 13 die *in uterus*. If survived, the clinical features include mental retardation, microcephaly and holoprosencephaly, structural eye defects, and congenital cardiac anomalies.

Patau K et al. Multiple congenital anomaly caused by an extra autosome. *Lancet* 1960; **1**: 790–793.

13. C. Heritability is the proportion of variation in a trait that can be attributed to genetic factors. It does not apply to a specific trait in an individual patient; it refers to the variation in the population as a whole. It is not immutable for a specific disease in a population; it will vary with the epidemiological changes in risk and environmental influences in a population, but it can be fixed at a specific time and for a given set of circumstances. Heritability is related to the feasibility of finding a candidate gene for a disease or trait; if a disease has zero heritability in a population, there is no chance of finding a gene. But this *does not* mean that 'the higher the heritability, the greater the feasibility of locating the genetic cause'. Heritability can be measured for polygenic disorders even when candidate genes are not known.

The phenotypic variation seen in the general population for a particular trait, say height of a person, can be explained by:
1. Total environmental effects—includes both shared and non-shared environmental effects
2. Total genetic effects—includes both additive genetic effects and dominance effects.
Narrow-sense heritability refers to the proportion of total phenotypic variation that can be attributed to additive genetic variance. The proportion of the total phenotypic variation attributed to total genetic variance is called broad-sense heritability.

Kendler K. Psychiatric genetics: a methodologic critique. *American Journal of Psychiatry* 2005; **162**: 3–11.

14. D. The risk of severe affective disorder in first-degree relatives of probands with bipolar disorder is 19%. The average morbid risk of bipolar disorder itself is 8%, while unipolar depression is around 11% in the first-degree relatives of probands with a bipolar disorder. The risk of severe affective disorders in first-degree relatives of probands with unipolar depression is estimated to be around 10%. Note that the lifetime risk of severe affective illness is about 3 to 5% for unipolar and 1% for bipolar disorders in the general population.

Scourfield J and McGuffin P. Familial risks and genetic counselling for common psychiatric disorders. *Advances in Psychiatric Treatment* 1999; **5**: 39–45.

15. A. The clinical description in the question fits with cri-du-chat syndrome. This is a result of partial deletion of small arm of chromosome 5. Cri-du-chat syndrome was first described by a French paediatrician, Lejeune, in 1963; he coined the term 'cri-du-chat' (cry of the cat). The commonly associated clinical features of cri-du-chat syndrome are:
1. Cat-like cry
2. Dysmorphic facies
3. Profound global learning disability.
It is now recognized that this triad does not present in all patients. Restrictive language skills and severely delayed psychomotor development are other notable features.

Cornish K and Bramble B. Cri du chat syndrome: genotype–phenotype correlations and recommendations for clinical management. *Developmental Medicine and Child Neurology* 2002; **44**: 494–497.

16. B.   COMT polymorphism has been widely studied in schizophrenia. COMT stands for catechol-o-methyl transferase. It is an important enzyme in the breakdown of dopamine in prefrontal area of the brain. Though monoamine oxidase is the major enzyme in dopamine metabolism in most other brain regions, COMT assumes special significance in the prefrontal brain area, at least in primates; the dopamine (reuptake) transporter is present at a low density in the prefrontal area compared to the striatum. The gene for COMT is located on chromosome 22q11. The deletion of 22q11 results in velo cardio facial syndrome (VCFS) or di George syndrome. As many as 30% of affected individuals with VCFS meet diagnostic criteria for schizophrenia. The existence of a valine-to-methionine (Val/Met) polymorphism has been noted, stimulating more interest in COMT. Val/Val genotype results in a higher activity form, while Met/Met is associated with lower activity of the enzyme. The higher activity variant leads to faster breakdown and reduced availability of prefrontal dopamine. This may be associated with poorer working memory function or inefficient prefrontal activity in such tasks.

Findings implicating GABA in working memory have been reported. Decreased expression of the GABA biosynthetic enzyme glutamic acid decarboxylase 67 (GAD67), encoded by *GAD1*, is found in the post-mortem brain tissue of schizophrenia patients. It has been shown that the variation in *GAD1* influences multiple domains of cognition, including declarative memory, attention, and working memory. There may be epistasis between SNPs in *COMT* and *GAD1*, suggesting a potential biological synergism, leading to increased risk. These coincident results implicate *GAD1* in the aetiology of schizophrenia and suggest that the mechanism involves altered cortical GABA inhibitory activity in addition to COMT changes (Straub *et al.* 2007).

Williams HJ *et al.* Is *COMT* a susceptibility gene for schizophrenia? *Schizophrenia Bulletin* 2007; **33**: 635–641.

Straub RE, Lipska BK, Egan MF *et al.* Allelic variation in GAD1 (GAD_{67}) is associated with schizophrenia and influences cortical function and gene expression. *Molecular Psychiatry* 2007; **12**: 854–869.

17. A.   Chemical modification of DNA is one method by which gene expression is controlled. This can be achieved by adding methyl groups to some of the amino acids in DNA. In females, randomly picked X chromosomes undergo methylation (Lyon's hypothesis) resulting in Barr bodies. In fragile-X syndrome, the fragile X site undergoes methylation, resulting in reduced expression of the *FMR1* gene on X chromosomes. This produces the phenotype of fragile-X syndrome. Unwinding of DNA is an important step that precedes DNA synthesis (replication from the template). Crossing over, condensation, and uncoiling are seen in the normal cell cycle. Genes do not become inactivated during such processes and subsequent cellular synthetic processes are intact.

Adams RLP. DNA methylation: The effect of minor bases on DNA-protein interactions. *Biochemical Journal* 1990; **265**: 309–320.

18. A.   In genomic imprinting, the disease phenotype expressed depends on whether the allele is of maternal or paternal lineage. This parent-of-origin phenomenon is an important exception to Mendelian inheritance patterns. An often-quoted example is Angelman's syndrome and Prader–Willi syndrome. These are two clinically distinct, genetic diseases associated with genomic imprinting on chromosome 15q11-q13. Major diagnostic criteria for Prader–Willi syndrome include mental retardation, hypotonia, hyperphagia and obesity, hypogonadism, and maturational delay. In Angelman's syndrome ataxia, tremors, seizures, hyperactivity, and profound mental retardation are accompanied by outbreaks of laughter (gelastic attacks). Approximately 70% of patients with Prader–Willi syndrome have a deletion in their paternally derived 15q11-q13. Maternal uniparental disomy (inheriting both copies from the mother when the embryo is formed) occurs in most of the remaining patients (25%). Most patients with Angelman's syndrome have a deletion in their maternally derived 15q11-q13. Paternal uniparental disomy occurs in about 4% of Angelman's syndrome. This parent-of-origin effect is thought to be due to DNA methylation defects.

Genetic anticipation refers to the phenomenon wherein phenotypic expression of a mutation occurs earlier in successive generations. This is seen in Huntington's disease and other trinucleotide repeat diseases. Autosomal aneuploidy, such as Down's syndrome, are not 'inherited' diseases but show a correlation with maternal age, as an ageing ovum is prone to more cell division errors. This is not the same as the parent-of-origin effect.

Falls JG et al. Genomic imprinting: implications for human disease. American Journal of Pathology 1999; **154**: 635–647.

19. C.   The anticipation phenomenon refers to an aspect of several genetic disorders in which the age at onset decreases and the severity of illness increases in successive generations. The classical example is Huntington's disease. This is also noted in other trinucleotide repeat syndromes. Trinucleotide repeats undergo expansion during germ cell division, which further destabilizes the mutant trinucleotide loci and the probability of the phenotypic expression thus increases with every gametogenesis. This occurs more frequently with oogenesis than spermatogenesis, leading to pronounced anticipation in maternally transmitted trinucleotide diseases. Carriers of a heterozygous recessive mutation may show cellular level abnormalities lifelong without overt disease manifestation; this is not genetic anticipation.

McGuffin P et al., eds. Psychiatric Genetics and Genomics. Oxford University Press, 2002, pp. 19–20.

20. C.   This description refers to MELAS, which shows mitochondrial inheritance. In mitochondrial inheritance, the disease is transmitted from females to males but not from males to females. MELAS stands for mitochondrial myopathy, encephalopathy, lactic acidosis, and recurrent stroke. MELAS is a progressive neurodegenerative disorder. Patients may present with seizures, diabetes mellitus, hearing loss, short stature, and exercise intolerance.

Leonard JV and Shapira AHV. Mitochondrial respiratory chain disorders I: mitochondrial DNA defects. Lancet 2000; **355**: 299–304.

21. D. In testicular feminization syndrome, the karyotype is usually 46 XY. Due to insensitivity of androgen receptors, female sexual characteristics develop in such individuals. They will not have Barr bodies. In those with Kleinfelter's syndrome, the karyotype is usually 47 XXY. Here, the individuals will have one Barr body in spite of being phenotypical males. Patients with Turner's syndrome have no Barr bodies as they have only one X chromosome, in spite of being phenotypical females. Patients with triple-X syndrome show two Barr bodies in each cell. These individuals are also called metafemales. In fragile-X syndrome the number of Barr bodies will not be altered.

Barr ML and Bertram EG. A morphological distinction between neurones of the male and female, and the behaviour of the nucleolar satellite during accelerated nucleoprotein synthesis. *Nature* 1949; **163**: 676–677.

22. A. Premutation is a term used in trinucleotide repeat diseases to suggest that someone is harbouring the trinucleotide expansion but the expansion is not long enough to produce the disease. But premutants will produce further expansion of the loci during gametogenesis and thus their children will express the mutation if inherited. In this question the mother has no phenotypic expression, which is rare to occur after age 32. Her genotype cannot be normal as her uncle and son are both affected by fragile-X syndrome. Fragile-X syndrome has nearly complete penetration falsifying the fourth option.

Jacquemont S, Hagerman RJ, Leehey M *et al.* Fragile X premutation tremor/ ataxia syndrome: molecular, clinical, and neuroimaging correlates. *American Journal of Human Genetics* 2003; **72**: 869–878.

23. A. The mother has genotype pp. Her gametes can both have p only. The father has Pp. His gametes may be either p or P. If these gametes combine in the children four possible combinations—pp, pp, pP, and pP—will be produced. Hence there will be 1/2 pp and 1/2 Pp variants in the children.

Kumar PJ and Clark ML. *Clinical Medicine*, 6th edn. Elsevier, 2006, p. 182.

24. E. This question refers to Edwards' syndrome, which is 18 trisomy. This is an aneuploidy. Euploidy refers to the presence of chromosomal numbers in multiples of 23. Haploid refers to the presence of 23 chromosomes, as normally seen in gametes. Most somatic cells are diploid, possessing 46 chromosomes. Aneuploidy refers to any aberrations in chromosomal numbers, for example monosomy, trisomy, etc. Edward's syndrome is characterized by 47XX +18 or 47XY +18 constitutions. It is seen in around 1 in 6000 live births; 90% of infants die in the first year of life. The common clinical features are small size, small mouth and low-set ears, clenched fist with overlapping fingers, congenital heart defects, and omphalocele.

Edwards JH, Harnden DG, Cameron AH *et al.* A new trisomic syndrome. *Lancet* 1960; **1**: 787–790.

25. B. Angelman's syndrome is an example of genomic imprinting. Deletion of maternally inherited 15q11-13 (70%) or uniparental disomy where both 15q11-13 come from the father (4%) leads to Angelman's syndrome. This is because certain genetic loci in 15q11-13 are selectively imprinted (that is inactivated via methylation) according to the parent of origin. When the maternally derived chromosome is absent due to deletion or paternal disomy this produces the phenotype. Similarly, maternally derived disomy or deletion of the paternally derived chromosome can produce Prader–Willi syndrome at the same locus.

McGuffin P *et al.*, eds. *Psychiatric Genetics and Genomics*. Oxford University Press, 2002, p.17 and p. 20.

26. D.   This question tests one's knowledge of the Hardy–Weinberg equilibrium. In a large population where random mating occurs between individuals, a constant and predictable relationship exists between various genotype and allele frequencies. If the frequency of an allele, A, is given by p, then at the same locus a second allele, B, has a frequency q = 1 − p. The frequency of AA individuals is given by p × p = p^2. The frequency of BB is thus q^2. The frequency of heterozygosity is given by 2pq as the heterozygosity can be AB or BA, both denoting the same constitution. According to the Hardy–Weinberg equilibrium $p^2 + 2pq + q^2 = 1$. This is true because $(p + q)^2 = (p + 1 − p)^2 = 1^2 = 1$. Note that deviations from the Hardy–Weinberg equilibrium can occur due to assortative non-random mating, natural selection, genetic drift, or gene flow.

McGuffin P *et al.*, eds. *Psychiatric Genetics and Genomics.* Oxford University Press, 2002, p. 39.

27. C.   An endophenotype is an unseen but measurable phenomenon that is present in the distal genotype to disease pathway. It can be a biochemical, neuroimaging, electrophysiological, pathological, neuropsychological, or sociofunctional marker. To be termed an endophenotype, Gottesman suggested certain criteria to be satisfied by an identified disease marker. These are as follows:
1. Must be associated with a candidate gene or region
2. Must be present with a high relative risk in relatives, thus co-segregating with the actual illness
3. Must be a parameter associated with the disease with biological plausibility
4. Must be expressed independently of clinical state (i.e. must not be a state but a trait marker)
5. Must be heritable
6. Must be present in relatives more often than the general population.

Gottesman II and Gould TD. The endophenotype concept in psychiatry: etymology and strategic intentions. *American Journal of Psychiatry* 2003; **160**: 636–645.

28. A.   Reciprocal translocation refers to exchange of genetic material between two chromosomes. An individual who carries a reciprocal translocation will not be affected clinically as he or she will have the normal complement of all essential genetic material. However, the children of such an individual can inherit partial trisomy or partial monosomy of the translocated chromosomes. Robertsonian translocations occur in approximately 1 in 1000 individuals. This refers to the loss of short arms of two acrocentric chromosomes (which do not have much genetic material) and subsequent fusion of the two chromosomes at 'sticky' centromeres. Again there is no effect in the individuals who suffer such a translocation but their children can inherit the effects. Five per cent of Down's syndrome children have inherited a Robertsonian translocation between chromosome 14 and 21, leading to triple copies of chromosome 21. In a mother with a 14:21 translocation, the risk of subsequent children having Down's syndrome is elevated to 10–15%, irrespective of maternal age. The risk is around 1–2% if the father carries such a translocation. Note that in a mother less than 30 without a translocation who has given birth to a Down's syndrome baby, the chances of recurrence is only 1%. Inversion refers to a segment of chromosome between two breaks undergoing reinsertion into the same chromosome but in a reverse order. If these breaks occur on either side of a centromere, it is called pericentric inversion. If not, it is termed paracentric inversion. Duplication occurs during formation of chromatids, where more than two sister chromatids are created. Isochromosomes occur when chromosomes divide at a horizontal instead of vertical axis during cell division. Hence daughter chromatids will have two copies of the same arm of a chromosome. This is usually lethal for most chromosomes except the X chromosome, whose isochromosomes can result in Turner's syndrome in individuals who inherit isochromosome Xq (long arm). This indicates that most determinants of Turner's syndrome reside in the short arm of the X chromosome.

Kumar PJ and Clark ML. *Clinical Medicine*, 6th edn. Elsevier, 2006, p. 174.

29. D. Monogenic diseases follow single gene–single disease inheritance, as for example in phenylketonuria. However, the most common cause of genetic disorders is thought to be multifactorial or polygenic inheritance. Polygenic diseases are genetic disorders caused by mutations or changes in more than one genetic locus, for example neurofibromatosis can be caused by NF-1 or NF-2 mutations. When environmental factors also play a role in the development of a disease or trait, the term multifactorial is used to refer to the additive effects of many genetic and environmental factors. Multifactorial illnesses, for example diabetes, coronary heart disease, and possibly most psychiatric illnesses, are simultaneously influenced by multiple genes and by environmental factors.

Kumar PJ and Clark ML. *Clinical Medicine*, 6th edn. Elsevier, 2006, p. 173.

30. B. If both parents are heterozygous the chance that the child inherits an autosomal dominant disease is 3/4, that is 75% (out of four children, one may have both normal alleles, one may have both abnormal alleles, and two may have heterozygous make-up). With 75% penetrance, the chances of a child being affected reduces to 75% of the original chance. So 75% × 75% = nearly 57% will be affected. This means that the likelihood of having an unaffected child increases from 25 to nearly 40%. Hence, the lower the penetrance, the higher the likelihood of having an unaffected child. This does not depend on the sex or birth order.

Kumar PJ and Clark ML. *Clinical Medicine*, 6th edn. Elsevier, 2006, p. 169.

31. C. Gregor Johann Mendel was a monk who was interested in horticulture and botany. He studied garden peas and proposed 'laws' of inheritance. The first law is the law of uniformity. According to this law, if two plants that differ in just one trait (black and white) are crossed, then the resulting hybrids will be uniform in the chosen trait (either black or white, not blue). This is not entirely true as later geneticists demonstrated intermediate phenotypes resulting from codominant heterozygous expression. The second law is the principle of segregation. It states that for any particular trait, the pair of alleles of each parent separate and only one allele passes from each parent to an offspring. Which allele in a parent's pair of alleles is inherited is a matter of pure chance. For example if there are two alleles with one determining white colour and one determining black colour in the first generation, then these two alleles segregate and only one of them from each parent could be passed on to the second generation. This was later proved to be true by studying chromosomes during cell division. The third principle is the principle of independent assortment. It states that different pairs of alleles are passed to offspring independently of each other. The result is that new combinations of genes present in neither parent are possible. As a very simplistic example, if a man with blue eyes and brown hair fathers a child with a woman with brown eyes and black hair, their offspring can have blue eyes and black hair. The inheritance of blue eyes does not take brown hair 'with it'; these traits are independently assorted. Thus Mendelian principles are applicable to human genetics as well. Note that all traits studied using Mendelian genetics refer to categorical, all-or-none, traits, that is black vs. brown, blue vs. brown, tall vs. short, etc. It does not apply with the same simplicity to dimensional traits such as IQ or blood pressure.

McGuffin P *et al.*, eds. *Psychiatric Genetics and Genomics*. Oxford University Press, 2002, p. 37.

32. B.   Autosomal recessive traits skip generations and may 'catch families unaware'. Assuming a good degree of penetrance, an autosomal dominant pattern affects all generations. Mitochondrial diseases will affect all generations but via maternal inheritance. X-linked recessive disorders can skip generations but not X-linked dominant. Autosomal recessive diseases are clinically expressed only in homozygous states. Most commonly, the homozygote is produced by the union of two heterozygous parents (carriers) who themselves will be unaware of harbouring such an allele. The recurrence risk in children born to such parents is 25%. If an affected homozygote marries a heterozygote the recurrence risk is 50%. Consanguinity (union between relatives) increases the likelihood of inheriting autosomal recessive diseases as related parents may have both inherited carrier status for the same disease from their common ancestor.

Kumar PJ and Clark ML. *Clinical Medicine*, 6th edn. Elsevier, 2006, p. 169.

33. B.   Mutation is a sudden, permanent, and heritable change in the DNA sequence. Changes in DNA may be transcribed to mRNA and translated to proteins, leading to disease expression. Point mutation refers to a single base change in DNA. Point mutations are usually substitutions, where one base is replaced by another. It is termed a transition if a purine is replaced by another purine or a pyrimidine replaced by another pyrimidine (e.g. A to G). It is called a transversion if a purine is replaced by a pyrimidine or vice versa (e.g. A to T). According to the effect on the triplet code, mutations could be a frame shift or in-frame. In frame-shift mutations, the deletion or insertion is not in multiples of three codons, for example a five-base deletion mutation. This leads to a shift in the triplet reading frame with variable results. In-frame mutation refers to changes occurring in multiples of three bases, with no disturbances in the reading frame. According to the effect of a mutation on the protein product, mutations could be silent, mis-sense, or nonsense. A silent mutation causes no change in the protein product—this is possible because a single amino acid is often coded by more than one triplet sequence. In a silent mutation one triplet sequence is replaced by a different sequence but without changing the amino acid sequence. In a mis-sense mutation, the new mutant codon specifies a different amino acid with variable effects on the final protein product, for example in haemophilia and sickle cell anaemia. In a nonsense mutation the new codon is UUA, UGA, or UAG, which signal 'stop' to the amino acid sequence, resulting in a non-functional protein. Point substitutions do not shift the reading frame; they often occur in non-coding regions and go unnoticed. Even in coding regions they are often silent or mis-sense mutations.

Kumar PJ and Clark ML. *Clinical Medicine*, 6th edn. Elsevier, 2006, pp. 176–177.

34. A.   Thymidine and folate deprivation are used in the demonstration of fragile sites in chromosomes. Cytogenetic techniques now available for the direct molecular identification of such fragile sites. Fragile-X syndrome, Huntington's disease, spinal muscular disease, and myotonic dystrophy are some of the disorders associated with fragile, trinucleotide expansions in chromosomes.

Glover TW. FUdR induction of the X chromosome fragile site: evidence for the mechanism of folic acid and thymidine inhibition. *American Journal of Human Genetics* 1981; **33**: 234–242.

35. E.   Duration of untreated psychosis (DUP) is not an endophenotype. Working memory defects, information processing defects such as prepulse inhibition, smooth pursuit defects, glial cell changes, and certain other putative neurocognitive markers are termed probable endophenotypes for schizophrenia. To be an endophenotype, a characteristic must be observable independent of clinical state and must be measurable in relatives at a higher degree than in the general population. By definition, DUP cannot be measured in those who are not having psychosis.

Gottesman II and Gould TD. The endophenotype concept in psychiatry: etymology and strategic intentions. *American Journal of Psychiatry* 2003; **160**: 636–645.

36. B. Locus heterogeneity refers to the existence of mutations in different chromosomal loci resulting in the same disease phenotype. It is an important clinical phenomenon when attempting to test for the presence of a carrier state or mutation for a specific disease. For example, early-onset Alzheimer's disease could be caused by presenilin 1 or 2 mutations or by β amyloid precursor mutations. These mutations occur in chromosomes 14, 1, and 21, respectively. (Pleiotropy and allelic heterogeneity are explained below.)

Malats N and Calafell F. Basic glossary on genetic epidemiology. *Journal of Epidemiology and Community Health* 2003; **57**: 480–482.

37. A. When ascertaining cases for genetic family studies it is possible to miss certain cases as the disease has not occurred as yet in some members of the family. For example if a disease presents at age 40 on average, and if the studied family has three 'normal' members aged 50, 30, and 18, there is still the possibility that the latter two may become 'cases' in the future. Various methods of age correction have been employed to ascertain the morbid risk precisely in such cases. Weinberger's weighted age method is a popular approach. Life tables can also be used for age correction. In most genetic disorders, birth order does not play a role in disease expression as each birth is an independent genetic event. Duration or severity of illness does not complicate the issues in most family studies.

McGuffin P et al. *Seminars in Psychiatric Genetics.* Gaskell, 1994, p. 31.

38. A. Epistasis is the term used to describe gene interactions. Epistasis specifically refers to interaction between alleles at different genetic loci. This interaction is evident in the protein production and function of the involved genes. It can occur at the same step or at different stages of the same biochemical pathway. Variable expression refers to the variation in the degree of phenotypic expression seen in certain genetic disorders. Some individuals carrying the phenotype may be severely affected while others will only be mildly affected. This may be due to the effect of environment on a phenotype, allelic heterogeneity (different mutations causing a phenotype, leading to variation in expressed severity), or epistatic influences (another genetic loci conferring protection against severe expression by modifying the biochemical pathway at a distant site). Incomplete penetrance refers to the phenomenon where some individuals with the disease genotype do not display any signs of the disease at all. If the number of obligate carriers of a genotype (individuals who possess a genotype) is 100, and the number showing disease expression is 80, then the penetrance rate is 80%. Codominance refers to simultaneous expression of two alleles at a chromosomal locus, for example AB blood group when one chromosome has genotype A and the other has genotype B.

Malats N and Calafell F. Basic glossary on genetic epidemiology. *Journal of Epidemiology and Community Health* 2003; **57**: 480–482.

39. A. Multifactorial diseases could be defined by a threshold model. Considering psychiatric disorders, the families of affected individual often show substantially higher risk than the general population. These disorders can be described as quasicontinuous as the affected portion (defined categorically) of the population can be differentiated as mild to severe in the spectrum (continuous dimensions). This could be described as having a continuously distributed liability to develop the disease that is inherited, while the actual expression is multifactorial. If the liability crosses a particular threshold then disease expression could occur. This liability distribution curve is shifted to the right if relatives of a patient are considered, as, for the given threshold, more affected individuals are found in the families than in the general population.

McGuffin P et al., eds. *Psychiatric Genetics and Genomics.* Oxford University Press, 2002, p.46.

40. B.   The odds ratio in most psychiatric genetic association studies are in the order of 1 to 2, the median being 1.3. This is insufficient to prove a genetic cause for most disorders. To demonstrate a more significant odds ratio, very large sample sizes are required; this methodological problem is being surmounted, at least partially, by meta-analyses that are providing evidence for the role of certain genes in psychiatric disorders. Non-contingent gene–disorder association refers to the fact that the relationship is not influenced by other factors such as environment or presence of other genes, that is not polygenic or multifactorial. But most psychiatric disorders do not follow non-contingent association models. The causal pathway from an identified genetic abnormality to actual disease expression is too complex and not fully explored in most known genetic markers of psychiatric diseases. For example it is unclear how a mutant dysbindin gene can lead to a belief that aliens are invading earth. There are few notable exceptions to this; for example the role of the serotonin transporter polymorphism in mediating the effects of life events on the risk of depression. For a long time, much genetic research was guided by the assumption that genes cause diseases, but the expectation that direct paths will be found from gene to disease has not proven fruitful for complex psychiatric disorders. Gene × environment interaction models of disease causation appear promising, as in Caspi's work, and may possibly throw more light on the causal chains from gene to disease.

Kendler KS. 'A gene for. . .': the nature of gene action in psychiatric disorders. *American Journal of Psychiatry* 2005; **162**: 1243–1252.

Caspi A *et al.* Influence of life stress on depression: Moderation by a polymorphism in the 5-HTT gene. *Science* 2003; **301**: 386–389.

41. A.   It has been demonstrated that the 'short' polymorphism in the promoter region of the serotonin transporter gene (*SLC6A4*) is associated with impaired efficacy of fluvoxamine and paroxetine. The long form is associated with better SSRI efficacy. This can be understood by studying the mechanism of action of SSRIs. SSRIs produce antidepressant action by reducing the activity of serotonin transporter protein. In patients with the short polymorphism of the promoter region, the number of serotonin transporter molecules is reduced, leaving less substrate on which SSRIs can act. Hence the short form is associated with poorer response than the longer form, but this might be confounded by an ethnicity effect as Korean and Japanese patients show the opposite effect (the short version is associated with better SSRI response).

Malhotra AK *et al.* Pharmacogenetics of psychotropic drug response. *American Journal of Psychiatry* 2004; **161**: 780–796.

42. C.   The name tuberous sclerosis comes from the characteristic tuber or potato-like nodules in the brain, which calcify and become sclerotic. The disorder is also known as epiloia or Bourneville's disease. Though most infants show signs in the first year of life, clinical features can be subtle initially, leading to misdiagnosis for years. The disease-causing mutations are present in either of two genes, *TSC1* and *TSC2*. *TSC1* is present on chromosome 9 and produces a protein hamartin. The *TSC2* gene is on chromosome 16 and produces a protein tuberin. The natural course is very variable, ranging from mild to severe illness. In addition to the benign tumours of kidney (cysts, angiomyolipomas), phakomas of eyes, cardiac tumours, and brain tumours (tubers, subependymal nodules, and astrocytomas) that frequently occur in tuberous sclerosis, other common symptoms include seizures, mental retardation, behaviour problems, and skin abnormalities. Malignant tumours are rare and occur primarily in the kidneys. An often quoted dermatological triad consists of adenoma sebaceum (facial angiofibromas), ash-leaf macules (hypomelanotic macules), and shagreen patches (pebbly skin on the nape of the neck). Café-au-lait patches and ungual fibromata are other manifestations of tuberous sclerosis. In most patients, tuberous sclerosis is due to a spontaneous new mutation but in those who inherit tuberous sclerosis, the pattern of inheritance is autosomal dominant.

McGuffin P *et al.*, eds. *Psychiatric Genetics and Genomics.* Oxford University Press, 2002, p. 117.

43. A. This description fits best with fragile-X syndrome. Fragile-X syndrome is also known as Martin–Bell syndrome. It is the most common cause of inherited mental retardation and is the second most common cause of genetically associated mental deficiencies after trisomy 21. Clinical features include mild-to-moderate autism-like behaviour, especially hand flapping and gaze avoidance, attention deficits, and learning disability with an IQ often in the range 35 to 70. Delays in reaching early milestones for speech and language developmental are also noted. Normally, unaffected individuals have 5 to 55 CGG repeats at the 5' end of locus Xq27.3. A span of 65–200 repeats is known as a premutation, whereas more than 200 repeats is a full mutation. Hypermethylation of cysteine bases takes place at the fully mutant locus, leading to gene inactivation. In trinucleotide expansion diseases, CAG expansion is seen in Huntington's disease (chromosome 4); CTG expansion is seen in myotonic dystrophy (chromosome 19).

McGuffin P et al., eds. *Psychiatric Genetics and Genomics.* Oxford University Press, 2002, p.119.

44. A. Allelic heterogeneity is said to be present if different alleles at the same locus produce the same trait or disease expression. Consider sickle cell disease. In this condition all affected individuals carry the same mutation at the same locus. This is called genetic homogeneity. But in cystic fibrosis, at the same site on chromosome 7, 600 various mutations have been identified that result in the same disease phenotype. This is called allelic heterogeneity. Locus heterogeneity refers to a single disorder, trait, or pattern of traits that is caused by mutations in genes at different chromosomal loci.

Gelder M et al., eds. *New Oxford Textbook of Psychiatry.* Oxford University Press, 2000, p. 247.

45. C. Pleiotropy is a very common phenomenon among genetic diseases. It refers to a single genetic defect producing a variety of defects, in multiple organs in the body, for example Marfan's syndrome. Here, an autosomal dominant mutation of a gene encoding fibrillin protein leads to a variety of defects, such as lens dislocation, skeletal deformities, and cardiac defects, especially aortic vessel disease.

Pyeritz RE. Pleiotropy revisited: molecular explanations of a classic concept. *American Journal of Medical Genetics* 2005; **34**: 124–134.

46. A. This refers to a frame-shift mutation. When a mutation results in misreading of a single triplet while other consecutive triplets are read correctly, it is called an in-frame mutation. If a mutation (usually a deletion or insertion) results misreading of all subsequent codons, then it is termed a frame-shift mutation.

Kumar PJ and Clark ML. *Clinical Medicine*, 6th edn. Elsevier, 2006, p. 176.

47. B. According to the law of segregation, inheritance of one trait occurs independently of another trait, but this is not always the case. This is due to random crossing over during meiosis, which allows the exchange of genetic segments that are significantly longer than a single gene. Such a crossing over results in the recombination of distant genetic loci. When two loci are close together, recombination is very unlikely and they are inherited as a single genetic element at a frequency significantly more than chance. This is called cosegregation, and the loci are said to be linked. Note that an essential condition for linkage is that the two loci must be on the same chromosome, called as syntenic loci; but not all syntenic loci are linked. Study of such linked loci is called linkage analysis. Restriction fragment length polymorphism is a method of genotyping single nucleotide polymorphisms using restriction endonucleases. Fluorescent *in situ* hybridization (FISH) involves denaturation of DNA on microscope slides and binding of sequence-specific DNA probes to the regions of interest on the exposed DNA strands. It is often used to study areas of deletion in chromosomes.

McGuffin P et al., eds. *Psychiatric Genetics and Genomics.* Oxford University Press, 2002, p. 55.

48. D. The distance between two loci can be measured in terms of the frequency with which they undergo recombination. For linked loci the frequency of recombination is less than 50%. Genetic distances are often expressed in centiMorgans (cM). One cM is equal to 1% recombination frequency between two loci, which can occur if nearly one million base pairs separate the two loci. LOD scores (log of odds) are used to estimate the likelihood that an observed recombination frequency is truly due to the loci being linked. It is given by the log of the ratio between the probabilities of the recombination frequency being the observed value (θ) to the expected value of 50% if they are not linked. A LOD of more than 3 indicates a linkage; less than −2 indicates no linkage. The value of θ at which LOD scores are greatest is the most likely estimate of recombination frequency.

Malats N and Calafell F. Advanced glossary on genetic epidemiology. *Journal of Epidemiology and Community Health* 2003; **57**: 562–564.

49. C. LOD scores were first used by Morton in 1955. It is a statistical method to establish linkage disequilibrium. A LOD (or log of odds) score is the common log of the likelihood that the recombination fraction has a certain value, θ, divided by the likelihood that it is 1/2. Conventionally, a LOD of 3, representing an odds of linkage of 1000: 1, is the accepted level for concluding linkage.

Malats N and Calafell F. Advanced glossary on genetic epidemiology. *Journal of Epidemiology and Community Health* 2003; **57**: 562–564.

50. C. Genotype frequency measures the proportion of each genotype, AA or AB or BB, in a population. Gene frequency measures the frequency of each allele at a particular locus in the population. Here, the frequency of allele A is $(40 \times 2) + 54 = 134\%$ or 1.34. The frequency of B is $(6 \times 2) + 54 = 66\%$ or 0.66.

Kumar PJ and Clark ML. *Clinical Medicine*, 6th edn. Elsevier, 2006, p. 190.

51. A. Consider an epileptic disease with generalized tonic–clonic seizures which could be caused by a genetic alteration. An identical generalized seizure could be a result of head injury that someone sustained. This is called as phenocopy. Here, phenotypic expression occurs in the absence of a genotype, due to a non-genetic reason. The term pleiotropy and the two types of heterogeneity—allelic and locus—are explained elsewhere in this chapter.

Malats N and Calafell F. Basic glossary on genetic epidemiology. *Journal of Epidemiology and Community Health* 2003; **57**: 480–482.

52. E. Gene frequencies and genotype ratios in a randomly breeding population remain constant from generation to generation. This is known as the Hardy–Weinberg law. This holds true only if the population is randomly breeding. If mutations are occurring in two genes at different frequencies, then this does not hold true as gene frequencies would change. In addition, if members of one population breed with occasional immigrants from an adjacent population this will introduce new genes or alter existing gene frequencies in the population. This is called gene flow. Similarly, strong interbreeding can happen within members of local populations. If the population is small, the Hardy–Weinberg equilibrium may be violated. As random mating can be assured only if sufficient numbers of matings occur, this is not possible in a small population. In such cases, the frequency of an allele may begin to drift toward higher or lower values. This is called genetic drift; it is accidental and aimless and is not an adaptive genetic change as it does not guarantee that the new generations will be more fit than the predecessors. In natural selection, certain alleles are positively selected and so their frequencies increase compared to other genes. This will result in failure of the Hardy–Weinberg equilibrium.

Malats N and Calafell F. Basic glossary on genetic epidemiology. *Journal of Epidemiology and Community Health* 2003; **57**: 480–482.

53. C. RNA is produced from DNA via transcription in most eukaryotic cells. A reverse procedure, where DNA is produced from RNA, takes place in certain viruses, especially retroviruses, including HIV. This procedure is mediated by a reverse transcriptase enzyme. DNA ligase acts in sealing DNA ends together during DNA replication. RNA polymerase acts in transcription of RNA from DNA. Primase acts in the initiation of DNA synthesis by catalysing the synthesis of RNA primers; this is necessary because DNA polymerases cannot initiate DNA synthesis without the help of RNA primers. When DNA replication is complete, DNA polymerase 1 destroys the RNA primers. DNA polymerase 1 contains an exonuclease which helps in proof-reading activity during DNA synthesis.

Kumar PJ and Clark ML. *Clinical Medicine*, 6th edn. Elsevier, 2006, p. 165.

54. C. Mitosis takes place in six identifiable phases. During interphase a cell is at rest. The individual chromosomes are not visible and active growth takes place. During prophase, which is the first phase of mitosis, the chromosomal material doubles and the nuclear membrane is broken down. Centrioles and spindle fibres become visible. During metaphase the chromosomes are equatorially aligned. Each centromere is now attached to two spindle fibres coming from opposite poles. During anaphase, the chromosomes separate and travel to opposite poles. During telophase an indentation appears in the cellular membrane and cytokinesis is then completed.

Morgan DO. *The Cell Cycle: Principles of Control*. New Science Press, 2007, p. 4–5.

55. A. In prophase, condensation of the replicated chromosomal material leads to the formation of sister chromatids, still attached at the centromeres. Each chromosome has two short and two long chromatids, corresponding to the short and long arms of the chromosomes.

Morgan DO. *The Cell Cycle: Principles of Control*. New Science Press, 2007, p. 4–5.

56. D. This can be calculated using the Hardy–Weinberg equilibrium. If p and q are the allele frequencies of recessive copy 'a' and dominant copy 'A', respectively, then p2 gives the frequency of homozygous aa and q2 gives the frequency of homozygous AA. 2pq gives the frequency of the heterozygous aA. 1/1600 is the frequency of homozygous individuals, that is p2. Hence, p = 1/40. If p = 1/40, then q will be 1 − p = 39/40. The number of heterozygous carries is given by 2 × 1/40 × 39/40 = 1/20 approximately. As one can see easily from this calculation, at any given time in a population there are more heterozygous carriers than diseased individuals. So negative eugenics, that is elimination of all diseased individuals, cannot eliminate an autosomal recessive disease.

Malats N and Calafell F. Basic glossary on genetic epidemiology. *Journal of Epidemiology and Community Health* 2003; **57**: 480–482.

57. E. Arachidonic acid is a fatty acid often found in membrane phospholipids. It is not a component of nucleic acids. Nucleic acids are made up of a purine or pyrimidine base, a pentose sugar moiety, and a phosphate group. Depending on whether the sugar is deoxyribose or ribose sugar, nucleic acids are either DNA or RNA.

Kumar PJ and Clark ML. *Clinical Medicine*, 6th edn. Elsevier, 2006, p. 164.

58. A. Association studies simply compare the frequency of a particular marker, for example a polymorphism, in diseased and normal populations. These are usually case–control studies and are comparatively easy to carry out. Linkage studies investigate the cosegregation of a disease and a set of genetic markers. Here, the aims are to determine linkage among candidate loci and determine the genetic distance between loci in an attempt to narrow down the site of the genetic abnormality. Linkage study is possible only if at least one parent has a double heterozygote make-up, that is heterozygous at both marker and disease loci. Family study refers to a genetic study whereby cases are ascertained by interviewing all available relatives of an identified proband. Age correction must be applied in such family-based case ascertainments. Adoption study investigates shared traits or phenotypes among adoptees, adopting families, and biological families in various combinations. Ecological study is not a specific genetic study.

Gelder M *et al.*, eds. *New Oxford Textbook of Psychiatry*. Oxford University Press, 2000, pp. 236 and 240.

59. A. In twin studies, case ascertainment and zygosity assignment is done initially. Later, concordance or discordance is measured to determine the heritability. This could be done by counting the proportion of the total number of concordantly affected twins among all pairs studied (pair-wise concordance) or by calculating the proportion of the number of affected twins among all cotwins studies (probands-wise concordance). The latter is possible if there is a twin register maintained with systematic ascertainment. Zygosity does not influence selection of the methods. Multifactorial diseases are commonly studied using twin studies by both methods.

Gelder M *et al.*, eds. *New Oxford Textbook of Psychiatry*. Oxford University Press, 2000, p. 236.

60. B. Autosomal recessive diseases often skip generations. The usual pattern of inheritance is from two heterozygous carriers, who are often unaware of their carrier status until their child is born homozygous with the disease. The chance of having an offspring with homozygous inheritance is 1 in 4; in other words, one affected child for every three unaffected children born (1: 3). This ratio becomes 1: 1 (50%) if one of the parents is homozygous and suffering from the disease.

Kumar PJ and Clark ML. *Clinical Medicine*, 6th edn. Elsevier, 2006, p. 183.

61. E. Increased death rate will not affect the number of genes or genotype distribution in a population directly. All the other options given can alter the Hardy–Weinberg equilibrium.

Malats N and Calafell F. Basic glossary on genetic epidemiology. *Journal of Epidemiology and Community Health* 2003; **57**: 480–482.

62. A. For continuous traits such as IQ, path analysis could be used in measuring heritability from concordance rates. The heritability $h2 = 2(RMZ - RDZ)$. Here monozygotic concordance is 0.86 and dizygotic concordance is 0.61. Hence, heritability is given by $2 (0.86 - 0.61) = 2(0.25) = 0.5$.

McGuffin P *et al.*, eds. *Psychiatric Genetics and Genomics*. Oxford University Press, 2002, p. 45.

63. E. Cystic fibrosis follows an autosomal recessive inheritance pattern. It is one of the most frequently occurring recessive gene mutation in Caucasian populations, with an estimated frequency of 1 in 30 carriers in the general population. Single-gene disorders usually follow the Mendelian pattern of inheritance; notable exceptions are mitochondrial diseases, trinucleotide expansion diseases, and genomic imprinting.

Kumar PJ and Clark ML. *Clinical Medicine*, 6th edn. Elsevier, 2006, p. 185.

64. C. Path analysis provides a diagrammatic approach to estimate the contribution of genetic and environmental factors in inheritance of a trait. The shared environment and shared genetic make-up are drawn to demonstrate the sources of resemblance between two siblings. Path coefficients are calculated for each connecting path between the sources and the siblings, and sum of these coefficients can provide a genetic correlation between the siblings.

Gelder M et al., eds. New Oxford Textbook of Psychiatry. Oxford University Press, 2000, p. 237.

65. B. The relative influence of genetic factors in defining the variance in a trait is expressed as heritability. If this is defined as the proportion of the total phenotypic variance attributable to additive genetic variance, then it is known as narrow-sense heritability. Heritability is also sometimes used to describe the proportion of variance explained by the total genetic variance (additive and non-additive genetic variance); here it is called broad-sense heritability. Non-additive genetic influences include phenomena such as epistasis (gene–gene interaction) and dominance effects, where presence of one gene mitigates the expression of other gene. A twin pair is said to be concordant when both cotwins have the same disease expression (or both are disease free). The pair can be discordant if one of them harbours a disease while the other does not. Due to the higher degree of genetic similarity among monozygotic twins, one would expect higher concordance between monozygotic twins compared to dizygotic twins if the disease being studied has a significant genetic component.

Gelder M et al., eds. New Oxford Textbook of Psychiatry. Oxford University Press, 2000, p. 235.

66. C. A linkage to chromosome 17 has been shown for a specific variant of frontotemporal dementing syndrome. This syndrome is now referred to as frontotemporal dementia with parkinsonism-17 (FTDP-17). The linkage region contains the gene for tau protein. tau pathology is noted in various other dementing syndromes, including Alzheimer's disease, where inappropriate hyperphosphorylation of tau is implicated in the production of neurofibril tangles.

Tasman A, Maj M et al., eds. Psychiatry, 3rd edn. John Wiley and Sons, 2008, p. 397.

67. D. HLA stands for human leukocyte antigens. These molecules are expressed on the surface of white blood cells to coordinate the immune response. DR and DQ are two different types of HLA molecules. Many different HLA 'subtypes' (DR1, DR2, DQ1, DQB1*0602) exist normally. HLA DR2 subtype has been linked to narcolepsy–cataplexy syndrome. African-American narcoleptic patients are frequently DR2 negative but they have a stronger association with another HLA gene allele, HLA-DQB1*0602.

Singh S, George C, Krygger M, and Jung J. Genetic heterogeneity in narcolepsy. Lancet, 1990; **335**: 726–727.

68. D. The gene for the MAO-A enzyme is located on chromosome X. In males a single X chromosome yields two dissimilar *MAOA* genotype variations: a high and a low activity variant. Females have two copies of the X chromosome, hence they can have three different levels of MAO-A activity: a high–high activity group (homozygous high), a low–low activity group (homozygous low), and a third, heterozygous group with low–high (mixed pattern). Caspi et al. (2002) studied MAO-A related genetic influences on the outcome of childhood maltreatment. They found out that high MAO-A activity exerts a protective influence against the development of antisocial outcomes (such as adolescent conduct disorder, violent episodes, etc.), especially in maltreated boys and to some extent in girls.

Caspi A, McClay J, Moffitt TE et al. Role of genotype in the cycle of violence in maltreated children. Science 2002; **297**: 851–854.

69. D. Milder forms of mania respond better to lithium than severe mania. Patients with classical features of mania respond better than those with schizoaffective presentation. On a similar note, dysphoric mania, mixed affective episodes, and rapid-cycling mania respond poorly to lithium treatment. Having a family history of bipolar illness is suggestive of good prophylactic response of lithium in relapse prevention; such an effect is not clearly demonstrated for the effects of lithium in treating acute mania.

Stein G and Wilkinson G, eds. *Seminars in General Adult Psychiatry*, 2nd edn. Gaskell, 2007, p. 33.

70. E. Friedreich ataxia (FRDA1) is caused by mutation in the gene encoding a protein called frataxin. The locus of the frataxin gene has been mapped to chromosome 9q. The most common molecular abnormality that affects the site of this gene is a trinucleotide repeat expansion of the triplet codon GAA in intron 1 of the frataxin gene. Another locus for Fredreich's ataxia has been mapped to chromosome 9p; it is called FRDA2.

Lynch DR, Farmer JM, Balcer LJ *et al*. Friedreich ataxia: effects of genetic understanding on clinical evaluation and therapy. *Archives of Neurology* 2002; **59**: 743–747.

71. C. First-degree relatives share 50% of their genes in common. This genetic relatedness reduces to 25% among second-degree relatives and 12.5% among third-degree relatives. The possible contribution of genetic factors for a disorder can be studied using the resemblance of disease risk across successive generations. A strong genetic contribution is suggested by a 50% decrement in disease risk with successive generations. If the risk decreases by more than 50% this suggests that the disease is either multifactorial with the possibility of significant gene–environment interaction or a more complex mode of genetic transmission. The ratio of the rate of the disorder in relatives to the population-based rate is commonly denoted by λ. This does not refer to linkage equilibrium. For diseases that are autosomal dominant in inheritance, λ tends to exceed 20; for complex multifactorial disorders, λ derived from family studies tends to range from 2 to 5.

Tasman A, Maj M *et al*., eds. *Psychiatry*, 3rd edn. John Wiley and Sons, 2008, p. 258.

72. D. The proportion of phenotypic variation attributable to genetic causes is referred to as heritability in the broad sense. The proportion attributable to non-genetic causes includes shared and non-shared environmental variance, gene–environment covariance, and interaction. The estimate of heritability for major depression from twin studies is around 0.37. The relative risks based on the existing adoption studies suggest that the familial recurrence cannot be attributed solely to shared environmental factors. The remaining 63% of variance is almost wholly attributed to environmental factors unique to the individual.

Tasman A, Maj M *et al*., eds. *Psychiatry*, 3rd edn. John Wiley and Sons, 2008, p. 260.

73. C. The apolipoprotein-E ε4 (*APOE ε4*) allele increases the risk of Alzheimer's disease in a dose-dependent fashion. The odds of developing Alzheimer's disease are 2.6–3.2 times greater in those with one copy, and nearly 15 times higher in those with two copies of the *APOE ε4*. A significant protective effect has been noted in those with *ε2/ ε3* genotype. The population attributable risk due to *APOE ε4* allele for Alzheimer's dementia is very high due to its high frequency of occurrence in the general population. *APOE ε4* can also increase the risk of vascular dementia.

Davidson Y, Gibbons L, Purandare N *et al*. Apolipoprotein E ε4 allele frequency in vascular dementia. *Dementia and Geriatric Cognitive Disorders* 2006; **22**: 15–19.

Tasman A, Maj M *et al*., eds. *Psychiatry*, 3rd edn. John Wiley and Sons, 2008, p. 263.

74. C. A gene on locus 13q34, called *G72*, codes for D-amino acid oxidase activator (DAOA). A series of initial studies have identified this genetic locus as potentially contributing to schizophrenia susceptibility. The D-amino acid oxidase is the only enzyme oxidizing D-serine. D-serine is an important coagonist for the NMDA glutamate receptor. Hence it is posited that the variations in the *G72* gene may influence the efficiency of glutamate gating at *N*-methyl-D-aspartate-type (NMDA) receptors, but some later studies have failed to replicate the earlier findings. *G72* has also been associated with depression in psychotic patients and also with bipolar disorder.

Boks MPM, Rietkerk T, van de Beek MH *et al.* Reviewing the role of the genes G72 and DAAO in glutamate neurotransmission in schizophrenia. *European Neuropsychopharmacology* 2007; **17**: 567–572.

75. B. Only a very small percentage (nearly 1.5%) of the human genetic code carried in DNA encodes proteins. This is because a large proportion of human DNA consists of long intron sequences, which are non-coding portions that get spliced out when transcription takes place. Hence, even when the complete sequence of a genome is known, mapping the functional genetic code will be difficult. A transcriptome is defined as all messenger RNA (mRNA) molecules transcribed from the DNA in a cell. The mRNA molecules act as 'mediators' between DNA codes and actual protein products. A transcriptome is not unique for a species or even for an individual; this is because what genes are transcribed in a cell depends on the kind of cell (e.g. WBCs, hepatocytes, epithelial cells) and what function is being carried out by the cell at that time. Hence, environmental influences or physiological needs will modify the transcriptome.

Ito C and Ouchi Y. Toward schizophrenia genes: Genetics and transcriptome. *Drug Development Research* 2003; **60**: 111–118.

76. B. The monozygotic concordance for simple Mendelian disorders is approximately 100%. This is because the penetrance is usually complete (though it may vary) in simple Mendelian disorders. In contrast, penetrance is incomplete in schizophrenia. Phenocopies of schizophrenia are very common; multiple organic and drug-induced states resemble schizophrenia. Locus heterogeneity in the same family is not a feature of simple Mendelian disorders affecting single loci. As the exact genetic localization of schizophrenia is still not certain, locus heterogeneity cannot be determined for schizophrenia, but given the multifactorial nature of schizophrenia, significant locus heterogeneity is very likely. Mendelian disorders need not necessarily present in childhood; many autosomal dominant disorders present clinically only in adulthood.

Kendler KS and Eaves L, eds. *Psychiatric Genetics.* Review of Psychiatry Series, American Psychiatric Publishing, 2005, p. 108.

77. A. The human genome is comprised of two sets of 23 chromosomes, one set inherited from each parent, and the DNA encodes 30 000 genes. Formerly, it was believed that genes were almost always present in two copies in a genome, but recently large segments of DNA of various sizes have been found to differ in copy number. Such copy-number variations (or CNVs) can lead to dosage imbalances in both functional (exons) and non-coding (introns) regions. As a result, many genes that were thought to occur in two copies per genome have now been found to be present in one, three, or even more copies.

Daar AS, Scherer SW, and Hegele RA. Implications for copy-number variation in the human genome: a time for questions. *Nature Reviews Genetics* 2006; **7**: 414.

78. D. Fragile-X patients have more than 200 CGG repeats in the 5' untranslated region of the fragile-X mental retardation 1 gene (*FXMR-1*). As in other trinucleotide repeat diseases, these expansions originate from phenotypically normal individuals who carry an intermediate number of unstable repeats (60 to 200). Normal individuals have 6 to 60 repeats. Even in carriers with premutation, longer repeats are observed to be more toxic than shorter, near normal ones. These carriers may show evidence of a neurodegenerative condition distinct from fragile X. The degree of toxicity increases with abundance of the transcript. CAG repeats are seen in Huntington's chorea.

Casci, T. Fragile X: a class of its own. *Nature Reviews Genetics* 2003; **4**: 758.

79. A. Genetic testing for Huntington's disease involves testing the person at risk for the presence of excessive DNA repeats that predict development of clinical features. The test cannot predict the age at which the onset of such symptoms could occur. Almost all patients carry a specific mutant gene at chromosome 4 and the inheritance has complete penetrance. Earlier genetic testing involved linkage analysis with only probabilistic estimates given to at-risk individuals. The tested individuals were given a risk estimate of less than 5% or greater than 95%, based on the results. Since 1993, direct identification of the trinucleotide expansion has been made possible, greatly increasing the accuracy of the test to nearly 100%. Being an autosomal dominant condition, the disease exhibits an all-or-none phenomenon; homozygotes are no more severely affected than heterozygotes. Prenatal testing is possible even when the at-risk parent has not had a test him/ herself. In this case, only the proportion of the parent's risk that is passed on to the fetus can be estimated; often this may not give sufficient information to decide on termination of pregnancies. The disease can occur in persons with apparently no positive family history, though this is extremely rare nowadays.

Myers RH. Huntington's disease genetics. *NeuroRx* 2004; **1**: 255–262.

80. A. This patient presents with neurofibromatosis type 1. Patients with neurofibromatosis can present with light-brown spots on the skin (café-au-lait spots), neurofibromas, freckling in the area of the armpit or the groin, hamartoma of the iris (Lisch nodules), optic glioma, and scoliosis. Many children with NF1 have larger than normal head circumference and may have congenital heart defects. They may have poor linguistic and visual–spatial skills, in addition to attention deficit hyperactivity disorder (ADHD). Most symptoms are notable before the age of 10. The genetic localization of *NF1* points to chromosome 17. The *NF1* gene codes for a protein called neurofibromin, which acts as a regulator of cell division in the CNS. A second type of neurofibromatosis is called NF2; the clinical presentation and genetic abnormality seen in NF2 are different from NF1. The gene responsible for NF2 has been identified on chromosome 22. The *NF2* gene product codes a tumour-suppressor protein called merlin.

DeBella K, Szudek J, and Friedman JM. Use of the national institutes of health criteria for diagnosis of neurofibromatosis 1 in children. *Pediatrics* 2000; **105**: 608–614.

1. **Which of the following refers to the incidence rate of dementia in a catchment area?**
   A. Number of patients with dementia during a specified time interval
   B. Number of newly diagnosed patients with dementia
   C. Ratio of the number of newly diagnosed patients with dementia during a specified time interval to the total population in the same area
   D. Ratio of the number of patients with dementia at a given time to the total population in the same area
   E. Number of newly diagnosed patients with dementia who are still surviving at the time of the survey

2. **In a National Comorbidity Survey carried out in the US, the proportion of the sampled individuals who ever manifested criteria of panic disorder in their lifetime was determined. This can be best described as which of the following?**
   A. Incidence
   B. Point prevalence
   C. Lifetime prevalence
   D. Lifetime morbid risk
   E. Period prevalence

3. **Using case records, the number of newly diagnosed cases of psychosis in south-east London was determined for a period of 33 years, between 1965 and 1997. To calculate incidence rate, which of the following is the most suitable denominator?**
   A. Total south-east London population in the year 1965 minus number of cases
   B. Total south-east London population in the year 1997
   C. Census of south-east London population aged more than 16 in the year 1981
   D. Census of south-east London population aged more than 16 in the year 1965
   E. Census of south-east London population aged more than 16 in the year 1997

4. **Which of the following equations gives the relationship between prevalence and incidence?**

    A. Prevalence = duration of disease × incidence rate
    B. Incidence rate = duration of disease × prevalence
    C. Prevalence = mortality rate × incidence rate
    D. Incidence rate = mortality rate × prevalence
    E. Prevalence = mortality rate × incidence × duration of disease

5. **A major cause of mortality in schizophrenia is cardiovascular problems. If a new class of antipsychotics with favourable metabolic profile that reduces cardiac risk is introduced, which of the following could happen?**

    A. Increase in incidence and prevalence of schizophrenia
    B. Increase in prevalence of schizophrenia, but reduced incidence
    C. Increased prevalence but unaffected incidence
    D. Reduction in both incidence and prevalence
    E. Both incidence and prevalence will remain unaffected

6. **Which of the following expresses an incidence rate measured for a subgroup of a population?**

    A. Crude mortality rate
    B. Lifetime prevalence rate
    C. Standardized mortality rate
    D. Specific mortality rate
    E. Survival rate

7. **Which of the following correctly expresses proportional mortality rate due to anorexia nervosa?**

    A. Number of anorexia-related deaths in a year/ total midyear population
    B. Number of anorexia-related deaths in a year/ total number of all cause deaths
    C. Number of anorexia-related deaths in a year/ total number of new cases diagnosed with anorexia in the same year
    D. Number of anorexia-related deaths in a year/ 1-year prevalence of anorexia
    E. Number of all cause deaths in a year/ number of anorexia-related deaths in the same year

8. **Which of the following is a major advantage in using standardized morality rate compared to crude mortality rate?**

    A. Comparisons between populations is easier with the standardized rate.
    B. True value of the number of deaths in a population is given by a standardized rate.
    C. Standardized rates can be expressed in meaningful units while crude rates do not have a specific unit for expression.
    D. Standardized rates provide an idea about cause of deaths in a population.
    E. The accuracy of measurement is increased by using standardized rates.

9. There are 65 suicides in a population of 1300 patients with schizophrenia. The rate 65/1300 refers to which one of the following?

   A. Proportional mortality rate
   B. Cause-specific mortality rate
   C. Case fatality rate
   D. Standardized mortality rate
   E. Crude mortality rate

10. Patients with undiagnosed subsyndromal hypomania have clinical characteristics closely resembling which one of the following diagnoses?

    A. Bipolar type 1
    B. Dysthymia with depression
    C. Depression with stimulant use
    D. Bipolar type 2
    E. Major depressive disorder

11. In major epidemiological studies, the mean time lag between onset and clinical treatment for major depressive disorder is determined to be around

    A. 3 months
    B. 3 weeks
    C. 3 years
    D. 13 years
    E. 3 days

12. Considering the epidemiology of major depressive disorder, which of the following is incorrect with respect to seeking treatment?

    A. Nearly half of men with depression do not get treated.
    B. Women seek treatment more often than men.
    C. Treatment is sought earlier in developed countries.
    D. Less than 20% of depressive episodes do not come to clinical attention.
    E. Earlier onset is associated with poorer treatment-seeking behaviour.

13. Major depressive disorder often coexists with personality disorders. Which of the following groups of personality disorders is most commonly associated with depression?

    A. Paranoid, schizotypal, and schizoid
    B. Histrionic, borderline, and antisocial
    C. Dependent and anxious avoidant
    D. Sadistic and narcissistic
    E. Obsessive compulsive and passive aggressive

14. Major depressive disorder often coexists with personality disorders. What is the proportion of patients with major depression and lifetime comorbidity of personality disorders in community samples?

    A. 10%
    B. 60%
    C. 75%
    D. 3%
    E. 30%

15. To estimate the number of homeless mentally ill patients, an initial survey was carried out in a defined area of central London and identified patients were registered. Six months later, another random sampling was carried out and using the identified proportion of previously registered homeless mentally ill, reliable population values were deducted. This method of epidemiological survey is best described as

    A. Capture–recapture study
    B. Cohort study
    C. Cross-sectional survey
    D. Audit
    E. Comorbidity survey

16. **Who first coined the term comorbidity?**

    A. Folstein
    B. Feinstein
    C. Einstein
    D. Bradford Hill
    E. Gauss

17. **Which of the following is the best estimate of the incidence of schizophrenia if a rigorous systematic review of various epidemiological studies to date is carried out?**

    A. 15 per 100 000
    B. 1 per 100
    C. 4 per 1000
    D. 7 per 1000
    E. 5 per 100 000

18. **The male to female risk ratio for developing schizophrenia is calculated to be which of the following values?**

    A. 1 : 1
    B. 1.4 : 1
    C. 3 : 1
    D. 1 : 2
    E. 4 : 1

19. The risk ratio for developing schizophrenia in migrants compared to a native population is

    A. 1 to 2.6
    B. 1.6 to 1
    C. 4.6 to 1
    D. 6 to 1
    E. 1 to 1

20. The probability of developing a disorder anytime throughout the life course of a birth cohort is called

    A. Lifetime prevalence
    B. Lifetime morbid risk
    C. Life expectancy
    D. Period prevalence
    E. Cumulative incidence

21. Which of the following could be estimated using the summation of age-specific incidence rate of schizophrenia throughout the average life expectancy of a population?

    A. Age-specific prevalence rate of schizophrenia
    B. Lifetime morbid risk of schizophrenia
    C. Lifetime prevalence of schizophrenia
    D. Cumulative incidence of schizophrenia
    E. Period prevalence estimate of schizophrenia

22. The male: female ratio for prevalence of schizophrenia is estimated to be

    A. 1 : 1
    B. 2 : 1
    C. 3 : 1
    D. 1 : 2
    E. 2 : 3

23. The lifetime morbidity ratio associated with schizophrenia is estimated to be

    A. 15 per 100 000
    B. 1 per 100
    C. 4 per 1000
    D. 7 per 1000
    E. 5 per 100 000

24. The population attributable fraction for seasonal birth in the incidence of schizophrenia is estimated to be around

    A. 30%
    B. 50%
    C. 2%
    D. 10%
    E. 6%

25. **The incidence rate of an illness varies widely across different countries. The prevalence measures, calculated at the same time, do not follow the same pattern of variation but are uneven. Which of the following could explain this disparity?**

    A. Different scales were used for measuring new and old cases
    B. Recall bias explains the high incidence rates
    C. Respondent bias explains the prevalence rates
    D. The risk factors for causation and prognosis are different
    E. The disease is a fatal condition

26. **The frequency of adults reporting lifetime presence of mental health problems in Europe is estimated to be around**

    A. 1 in 4
    B. 1 in 10
    C. 1 in 2
    D. 1 in 25
    E. 1 in 100

27. **Considering pathways of care in mental health, which of the following is not a major filter for help seeking?**

    A. Self-recognition of emotional difficulties
    B. Diagnostic ability of a general practitioner
    C. Acceptance rate at secondary care
    D. Occupational health initiatives at a place of employment
    E. In-patient admission facilities at local psychiatric services

28. **In epidemiological surveys across life span, the term persistence refers to which of the following?**

    A. Number of patients with lifetime prevalence who have 12 months prevalence
    B. Number of patients with 12 months prevalence who will develop chronic problems if followed up
    C. Number of patients with lifetime prevalence who spent more than 1/3 of life with the disease
    D. Number of patients with lifetime prevalence who spent more than 1/2 of life with the disease
    E. Number of patients with lifetime prevalence who are seeking health-care input

29. **Epidemiological catchment area study is one of the major surveys in psychiatric epidemiology. Which of the following instruments was used for clinical diagnosis in this survey?**

    A. Composite international diagnostic interview
    B. Diagnostic interview schedule
    C. Schedules for clinical assessment in neuropsychiatry
    D. Operational criteria checklist
    E. Revised clinical interview schedule

30. **Which of the following could explain the differential outcome for schizophrenia between developing and developed nations?**
    A. Economic differences
    B. Diagnostic differences
    C. Differential methods used in outcome measurement
    D. Difference in mode of onset of psychosis
    E. None of the above

31. **Which of the following was a WHO-sponsored survey of outcome in schizophrenia across different countries?**
    A. IPSS study
    B. DOSMeD study
    C. NEMESIS study
    D. DEPRES study
    E. ECA study

32. **According to results from the World Mental Health Survey Initiative, which of the following is true?**
    A. Developed countries have more mental health problems
    B. Severity of mental illness is not proportional to seeking treatment
    C. The unmet needs of mental health are equal across all countries
    D. The most common mental disorder globally is alcohol misuse
    E. Most patients who receive treatment have severe illness.

33. **In Europe, the age group with highest prevalence of mental health problems is**
    A. Over 65
    B. Under 16
    C. 18 to 24
    D. 25 to 34
    E. 35 to 50

34. **In any given year, the proportion of Europeans who receive antidepressants for their depression is estimated to be around**
    A. 20%
    B. 40%
    C. 60%
    D. 5%
    E. 90%

35. **Among people who experience panic attacks, which of the following is the most common presentation?**
    A. Agoraphobia with panic attacks
    B. Isolated panic attacks only
    C. Panic disorder
    D. Panic disorder with agoraphobia
    E. Physical disorder causing panic attacks

36. **The proportion of Europeans with mental health difficulties who have sought help from a psychiatrist within the last 1 year is estimated to be around**
    A. 20%
    B. 40%
    C. 60%
    D. 5%
    E. 90%

37. **The mean age of onset of panic disorder or agoraphobia is estimated to be around**
    A. 22 years
    B. 33 years
    C. 44 years
    D. 55 years
    E. 11 years

38. **Women outnumber men in prevalence of most anxiety disorders. Which of the following anxiety disorders is noted more commonly in men than women attending health-care services?**
    A. OCD
    B. Panic disorder
    C. Agoraphobia
    D. Social phobia
    E. Specific phobia

39. **Which of the following types of specific phobia often starts before the age of 10?**
    A. Blood injury phobia
    B. Space phobia
    C. Situational phobia
    D. Agoraphobia
    E. Animal phobia

40. In an epidemiological survey, mood state and functional impairment are recorded using a purpose-built scale. Which of the following can increase the reliability of such a questionnaire?
    A. Increasing the number of questions pertaining to each theme
    B. Giving more time to respond to questions
    C. Reducing the length of questionnaire to minimum
    D. Using two observers for self-rated scales
    E. Making the responses unstructured but descriptive

41. In the Stirling County Study of the prevalence of depression and anxiety, the questions used to diagnose depression in 1952 were modified in 1992. Which of the following best explains why this was done?
    A. The concept of depression changed in 40 years.
    B. Diagnostic schemes changed in 40 years, necessitating modification of questions.
    C. Vernacular terms used in describing depression changed over 40 years.
    D. Availability of treatment differed between 1952 and 1992.
    E. Severity of depression changed in 40 years.

42. Which of the following epidemiological studies suggested that lifetime prevalence of depression has remained unchanged over recent decades?
    A. National Comorbidity Survey, 1994
    B. Epidemiological Catchment Area Study, 1984
    C. Stirling County Study, 1992
    D. National Epidemiological Survey on Alcohol and Related Conditions, 2002
    E. National Comorbidity Survey Replication, 2002

43. The prevalence of hallucinatory experiences in healthy British respondents from community samples is estimated to be around
    A. 4%
    B. 11%
    C. 33%
    D. 19%
    E. 0.2%

44. A sample of healthy British community respondents was surveyed for self-reported psychiatric symptoms. Most respondents would rate themselves to have had which of the following symptoms?
    A. Hallucinations
    B. Hypomania
    C. Paranoia
    D. Thought insertion
    E. Strange experiences

45. In epidemiological surveys of preschool children, which of the following factors observed around age 3 of a child predicts behavioural difficulties by age 8?

   A. Mother being a house-wife
   B. More than two children in the household
   C. Maternal depression
   D. Deprived neighbourhood
   E. Physical health problems at age 3

46. Mental health and problem behaviours in a community sample of 10- to 11-year-old children were recorded in the Isle of Wight study in 1960. The prevalence of diagnosable psychiatric disorders in this study was approximately

   A. 6%
   B. 21%
   C. 1%
   D. 16%
   E. 30%

47. Which of the following statements regarding epidemiological surveys in child and adolescent mental health is true?

   A. Psychiatric disorders decrease with increase in age.
   B. Adolescents have more burden of psychiatric diseases than younger children.
   C. The marital relationship of parents influences the severity but not prevalence of psychiatric diagnoses.
   D. Parents and teachers have a high degree of agreement as to which child is having mental health problems.
   E. Most children diagnosed in community surveys were known to mental health services.

48. Questionnaires used in epidemiological surveys can be administered either by clinicians or trained non-clinicians. Which of the following is true about these instruments?

   A. The rate of psychiatric diagnoses is more when using clinician administered instruments.
   B. The rate of psychiatric diagnoses is the same irrespective of the type of instrument.
   C. High level of agreement exists between SCAN (clinician administered) and CIS-R (layperson administered).
   D. Clinician administered instruments are superior for screening purposes.
   E. Often a structured lay interview is followed by clinical diagnostic assessment for case ascertainment.

49. **With regard to surveys of suicidal ideation, the transition from ideas to plans or attempts occurs most frequently in which of the following time intervals?**

    A. Within 1 week of the ideation
    B. Within 1 month of the ideation
    C. Within 3 months of the ideation
    D. Within 1 year of the ideation
    E. Within 10 years of the ideation

50. **In epidemiological surveys of suicidal ideation, which of the following factors is not associated with increased suicidal ideation?**

    A. Being female
    B. Being uneducated
    C. Being unmarried or separated
    D. Age between 25 to 44
    E. Having a psychiatric diagnosis

51. **Which of the following terms refers to the number of new cases observed per person-year of observation?**

    A. Cumulative incidence
    B. Incidence volume
    C. Incidence density
    D. Incidence velocity
    E. Incidence ratio

52. **Which of the following is the main focus of the current (third) generation of epidemiological studies in mental health?**

    A. To measure prevalence of the mental-health burden
    B. To measure the specific prevalence of individual disorders
    C. To measure the attitude of populations towards mental health
    D. To measure the burden of care faced by mental-health administrations
    E. To identify causal factors for severe mental illnesses

53. **When unmet mental health-care needs in the UK are considered, which of the following is incorrect?**

    A. Nearly 10% of the population have unmet need for treatment of a psychiatric disorder.
    B. Most unmet needs could be managed by a general practitioner.
    C. Less than half of all potential needs are met by health-care services.
    D. Huge investment in secondary care is required to meet the unmet needs.
    E. Unmet needs can be assessed using the Camberwell Assessment of Needs scale.

54. What is the estimated prevalence of adult ADHD according to the World Mental Health Survey Initiative?

A. 3.4%

B. 1.4%

C. 34%

D. 14%

E. 8.4%

55. Which of the following measures the impact of premature mortality on a population?

A. Crude mortality rate

B. Disease-specific mortality

C. Disability-adjusted life years

D. Years of potential life lost

E. Infant mortality rate

56. Which one of the following studies estimated the differences in incidence of psychosis in different ethnic groups in the UK?

A. UK 700 study

B. PRiSM Psychosis study

C. ESEMeD survey

D. AESOP study

E. UK household survey

57. According to epidemiological studies on the elderly population, the prevalence of mental disorders is estimated to be around

A. 10%

B. 2%

C. 50%

D. 5%

E. 30%

58. Which of the following lifespan studies is secondary research of pooled data from epidemiological studies estimating the burden of psychopathology in an elderly population?

A. NEMESIS

B. DEPRES

C. EURO-DEP

D. Isle of Wight Study

E. Epidemiological Catchment Area Study

59. With regard to psychiatric epidemiological studies of postpartum women, which of the following is false?

   A. Postpartum depression has no specific causal factors.
   B. Postpartum depression is not a continuum of postpartum psychosis.
   C. The Edinburgh postnatal depression scale is a self-rated scale.
   D. Postpartum psychosis occurs following around 1 per 1000 live-births.
   E. The recurrence rate of postpartum psychosis is about 1 in 10 pregnancies.

60. Considering the epidemiology of suicide in mental health-service users, in which of the following age groups are suicide rates higher in women than men?

   A. Less than 16
   B. 16 to 24
   C. 25 to 34
   D. Greater than 70
   E. None of the above

61. A new rating scale for anxiety that is under evaluation has a sensitivity of 80% and specificity of 90% against the standard ICD-10 diagnosis. Which one of the following is correct?

   A. Out of 10 truly anxious patients eight will be correctly identified as anxious by the scale.
   B. Out of 10 truly anxious patients nine will be correctly identified as anxious by the scale.
   C. Out of 10 normal volunteers eight will be correctly identified as normal by the scale.
   D. Out of 10 people who test positive using the scale eight will have true anxiety.
   E. Out of 10 people who test negative using the scale four will have true anxiety.

62. Which of the following best describes a receiver–operator curve? It is often used to

   A. Decide the presence of publication bias
   B. Decide the optimal cut-off of a screening test
   C. Predict the likelihood of a negative result in diagnostic evaluation
   D. Measure the survival rates of inception cohorts
   E. Test the inter-rater reliability of a new instrument

63. A pilot develops acute manic episode while flying with 200 passengers. After nearly 2 hours of struggle by the rest of the crew, the flight is flown to safety. The 200 passengers are followed up for development of PTSD symptoms in the next 2 years. This study can be termed a

   A. Case–control study
   B. Cohort study
   C. Case series study
   D. Qualitative study
   E. Cross-sectional survey

64. From a nationwide, cross-sectional survey it was found that 8% of otherwise normal children experience auditory hallucinations by the age of 11. This 8% of the survey sample was followed up annually for next 20 years to detect incidence of schizophrenia. This group can be termed a/an

    A. Inception cohort
    B. Open cohort
    C. Retrospective cohort
    D. Random cohort
    E. None of the above

65. X is strongly associated with Y. A study investigates whether X causes Y. Which one of the following weakens the claim for a causal association between X and Y?

    A. Consistency of association between X and Y
    B. Dose–response relationship between X and Y
    C. X always precedes Y
    D. U, V, and W are well-established effects of X
    E. X and Y are biologically related phenomena

66. An astute old age psychiatrist wants to know the prevalence of dependent personality disorder among the elderly population in his catchment area. The most appropriate research method he will be employing is

    A. Case–control study
    B. Cohort study
    C. Case series study
    D. Qualitative study
    E. Cross-sectional survey

67. Regarding the risk factors for adolescent alcohol problems, which of the following accounts for high attributable risk?

    A. Externalizing symptoms in childhood
    B. Maternal alcohol consumption
    C. Poor school performance
    D. Lack of friends
    E. Being a single child

68. A new test being evaluated to predict treatment response in geriatric depression utilizes neuroimaging techniques. The overall results of the test are very close to that observed on longitudinal follow-up after treatment (gold standard) but individuals vary widely in the magnitude of the results produced. Which one of the following correctly describes the properties of this test?
    A. Precise and accurate
    B. Precise but not accurate
    C. Not precise but accurate
    D. Neither precise nor accurate
    E. Accurate and sensitive

69. The lifetime prevalence of OCD is estimated to be around
    A. 0.5–1%
    B. 1–2 in 1000
    C. 2–3%
    D. 8–10%
    E. 10–15%

70. The prevalence of diabetes is higher among people with schizophrenia. Which of the following statements is correct with respect to the association between diabetes and psychiatric disorders?
    A. Diabetes is two to four times more prevalent in schizophrenia.
    B. Patients with treatment-resistant schizophrenia are less likely to be screened for diabetes.
    C. There is an unusually low rate of family history of type 2 diabetes in schizophrenia patients.
    D. Rates of impaired glucose tolerance in drug-naïve first-episode schizophrenia is less than in the general population.
    E. Schizophrenia is the only mental disorder showing an established association with diabetes.

1. C. The incidence of a disease is defined as the number of 'new' cases diagnosed in a specified time interval for a specified size of population at risk. The midinterval population usually determines this population size. For example while calculating the incidence of a disease in 1 year, the comparison is made against the midyear population.

$$\text{Incidence in 2008} = \frac{\text{Number of newly diagnosed cases in 2008}}{\text{Mid 2008 population in an area}}$$

Incidence is a rate ratio, that is it is measured against time. It is not a mere number and it is usually expressed per 100 000 persons in a population, per year. The essential criterion is that the measure should indicate all new occurrences of a disease within the period of observation in an area, irrespective of whether the newly diagnosed patients are cured or dead within the period of observation itself. For an accurate measurement of incidence, two cross-sectional surveys must be carried out in the same population; one must be at the beginning of a defined period and the other at the end of the same period.

Sadock BJ and Sadock VA. *Kaplan and Sadock's Comprehensive Textbook of Psychiatry*, 8th edn. Lippincott Williams and Wilkins, 2004: 175.

2. C. Lifetime prevalence is the proportion of individuals in the population who have ever manifested a disorder, who are alive on a given day. This is ascertained by surveying a population cross-sectionally and finding out if they ever satisfied the criteria for a disorder in the past or at the present time. As one can observe, although this method is commonly used in epidemiological surveys, it is prone to recall bias. Lifetime morbid risk refers to risk of contracting a disease for each individual in a birth cohort if they live long enough to reach the average life expectancy of the population. This must be clearly differentiated from prevalence estimates. Prevalence is largely a population measure, while lifetime morbid risk is more close to an individual's chances of being diagnosed with an illness.

Saha S, Chant D, Welham J, and McGrath J. A systematic review of the prevalence of schizophrenia. *PLoS Medicine* 2005; **2**: e141.

3. C. Incidence is a ratio between the number of newly diagnosed cases within a specified time period in a population and the total number of people living in the area (total population). To be accurate, such comparisons must exclude those who are not at risk, though this is generally not done for non-infectious, non-epidemic diseases such as psychiatric illnesses. It is essential that the denominator and numerator are not mutually exclusive, that is the diseased group must be a part of the studied population. Hence, when measuring the incidence of psychosis, the population above the age of 16 is the relevant denominator. The year 1981 is the midinterval period between 1965 and 1997.

Boydell J, Van Os J, Lambri M *et al*. Incidence of schizophrenia in south-east London between 1965 and 1997 *British Journal of Psychiatry* 2003; **182**: 45–49.

4. A.   Prevalence is defined as the number of 'existing' cases in a specified population for a period of observation (either cross-sectional observation, called point prevalence, or longitudinal observation for a specified time, called period prevalence). The existing cases include all new cases and all cases diagnosed before the observation but still suffering from the disease, but existing cases excludes those who have been previously diagnosed but are now cured or dead. For illnesses that are significantly chronic (e.g. schizophrenia), prevalence will be higher compared to those illnesses that are acute and short lived (e.g. influenza), even if the incidence rates are comparable. Hence the simple expression

$$prevalence = incidence \times duration\ of\ illness$$

explains the relationship between incidence and prevalence.

Freeman J and Hutchison GB. Prevalence, incidence and duration. *American Journal of Epidemiology* 1980; **112**: 707–723.

5. C.   Certain factors can influence incidence and prevalence differently. For example if a new vaccine is developed to prevent an illness, both incidence and prevalence may come down. If a cure is developed for schizophrenia, incidence may not be affected but prevalence could drop. Similarly, if interventions are introduced to reduce mortality in chronic schizophrenia, then prevalence may paradoxically increase due to longevity of patients. This may not affect incidence rates directly.

Higginson IJ and Constantinin M. Epidemiology of symptoms in advanced illness. In: Max MB and Lynn J, eds. *Symptom Research: Methods and Opportunities*. http://symptomresearch.nih.gov/ tablecontents.htm (accessed 19.8.08).

6. D.   Mortality rates are a special type of incidence rates where 'death' is the defined 'case' of interest. Crude mortality rate is the ratio between number of deaths due to all cause in a population and total population size. Cause-specific mortality rate, for example alcohol-specific mortality, refers to the ratio between the number of deaths due to alcohol in a population and total population size. A standardized rate is a rate applicable to a hypothetical population with an adjusted variable, for example age. As population samples are heterogeneous, crude rates from one population may not be comparable to another population. For example suicide rates in inner London may not be comparable to rates in rural Yorkshire, as the working-age population may be higher in London, spuriously increasing suicide rates. Hence, standardized hypothetical populations are used on which observed rates from a population are applied and adjusted values are derived. These standardized values are easily comparable, but they are not subgroup incidence rates.

US Department of Health and Human Services. *Principles of Epidemiology*, 2nd edn. www2a.cdc. gov/phtn/catalog/pdf-file/Epi_Course.pdf (accessed 19.08.2008), p. 100.

7. B.   Proportionate mortality rate is a measure of the contribution of a disease to societal mortality burden. It is given by the ratio between deaths due to a specific cause and total number of deaths in a population. Case fatality rate is the ratio between the number of deaths due to a specific disease and number of persons affected by the disease in a population. It is a measure of the fatal severity of the disease studied. For example 15 patients out of 100 with anorexia will die due to its complications. Choice A refers to cause-specific mortality rate while choice D refers to case fatality rate.

US Department of Health and Human Services. *Principles of Epidemiology*, 2nd edn. www2a.cdc. gov/phtn/catalog/pdf-file/Epi_Course.pdf (accessed 19.08.2008), p. 100.

8.A. The true value of the number of deaths in a population is obtained using crude mortality figures. Both standardized and crude rates are expressed in the same units of incidence. Standardized rates are not the same as specific rates. Disease-specific rates can give an idea about cause of death in a population. Standardized rates increase comparability, not the accuracy of measurement of mortality in a population.

US Department of Health and Human Services. *Principles of Epidemiology*, 2nd edn. www2a.cdc. gov/phtn/catalog/pdf-file/Epi_Course.pdf (accessed 19.08.2008), p. 100.

9.B. This is an example of cause-specific (suicide is the cause) mortality rate in a population (number of schizophrenia patients). If the comparison is between the number of patients died with a diagnosis of schizophrenia and total number of patients at a given time interval, then this becomes case fatality rate for schizophrenia. If deaths due to suicides in a population with schizophrenia are compared with all-cause deaths in the same population then this will be proportionate mortality due to suicide. A 'case' of suicide cannot be identified alive, though patients who attempted suicides can be identified. So describing a 'case' fatality rate for suicide is meaningless. Nevertheless, method-specific case fatality can be derived for various modes of suicide attempts.

US Department of Health and Human Services. *Principles of Epidemiology*, 2nd edn. www2a.cdc. gov/phtn/catalog/pdf-file/Epi_Course.pdf (accessed 19.08.2008), p. 100.

10. D. In large epidemiological studies, a consistent 1.5% prevalence is quoted for bipolar disorders. It is unclear whether there is an over-inclusion of depressive disorders and under-diagnosis of bipolar type 2 disorder in these surveys. Hypomania, being positively appraised by patients themselves, is often missed in structured, non-clinician interviews. Angst *et al.*, in a 20-year-long prospective study, observed that patients with depression and clinically undiagnosed subsyndromal hypomania have similar risk factors, course, and outcome compared to bipolar disorder type 2.

Angst J, Gamma A, Sellaro R *et al.* Recurrence of bipolar disorders and major depression. A life-long perspective. *European Archive of Psychiatry and Clinical Neuroscience* 2003; **253**: 236–240.

11. C. According to NESARC (National Epidemiological Survey of Alcoholism and Related Conditions) the mean age of onset of depression is 30 years, the mean number of episodes in patients with lifetime major depressive disorder is five, and the mean age of treatment onset for depression is 33.5 years. This lag of around 3 years is noted in other community samples that studied treatment seeking for depression. It is currently unclear if untreated depression, as noted in population surveys, affects clinical outcome in long-term follow-up.

Hasin DS, Goodwin RD, Stinson FS *et al.* Epidemiology of major depressive disorder: Results From the National Epidemiologic Survey on Alcoholism and Related Conditions. *Archives of General Psychiatry* 2005; **62**: 1097–1106.

12. D. Nearly 40% of depressive episodes do not come to clinical attention even in developed nations (NESARC study). The World Mental Health Survey initiative organized by the WHO revealed that older generational cohorts of depressed people, men, those with earlier age of depression onset, and those who are living in developing compared to developed countries are poor seekers of treatment for depression. The situation is even worse for anxiety and substance-use disorders. An encouraging finding was that those with severe illness sought treatment more often than those with milder illnesses.

WHO World Mental Health Survey Consortium. Prevalence, severity, and unmet need for treatment of mental disorders in the World Health Organization World Mental Health Surveys. *JAMA* 2004; **291**: 2581–2590.

13. C. The most common comorbidities with depression in epidemiological surveys are alcohol use (>40%) and anxiety (>40%). It is noted that cluster C personality disorders, with the exception of obsessive compulsive personality disorder, show strong associations with lifetime major depression in large-scale community surveys. In Question 13, choice A refers to cluster A personality, choice B to cluster B, and choice C to two of the three cluster C personality disorders. Choice D includes disorders described in DSM IV but not clustered in any of the three groups.

Hasin DS, Goodwin RD, Stinson FS *et al*. Epidemiology of major depressive disorder: Results From the National Epidemiologic Survey on Alcoholism and Related Conditions. *Archives of General Psychiatry* 2005; **62**: 1097–1106.

14. E. It is important to note that the prevalence of personality disorders in those who attend psychiatric services or primary-care services are higher than community prevalence rates. The rate of personality disorders is recorded to be very high in institutions such as prisons and psychiatric hospitals providing long-term services. The prevalence of any personality disorder in community samples is estimated to be around 13% in the UK. The comorbid association of diagnosable personality disorder and depression was explored in NESARC study, which revealed 30% of depressed patients in the community have a comorbid personality disorder.

Hasin DS, Goodwin RD, Stinson FS *et al*. Epidemiology of major depressive disorder: Results From the National Epidemiologic Survey on Alcoholism and Related Conditions. *Archives of General Psychiatry* 2005; **62**: 1097–1106.

15. A. This is called capture–recapture technique. It is useful in estimating the size of a population that cannot be directly estimated as only a fraction is observable when using sampling techniques. Initially, a random sample from the population of interest is drawn (e.g. mentally ill homeless population). After registering these patients they are allowed to mix with the population (using a registration tag, they can be identified again). When complete mixture with the total population has occurred, a second random sample is drawn. From the prevalence of the registered patients in the second sample, the size of the total population may be calculated. This technique is being used in animal research to provide estimates of census of animals.

Burger H and Neeleman J. A glossary on psychiatric epidemiology. *Journal of Epidemiology and Community Health* 2007; **61**: 185–189.

16. B. The term comorbidity refers to the existence of two different diagnoses at the same time in an individual. In psychiatric epidemiology, comorbidity is a rule rather than exception. This high degree of comorbidity is partly due to the overlapping nature of diagnostic entities in psychiatry. Comorbidity in epidemiological research throws light onto possible aetiological underpinnings and meaningful outcome variables. Feinstein coined the term comorbidity. The various types of comorbidity are:
1. Episode (concurrent) comorbidity
2. Lifetime comorbidity
3. Coincidental comorbidity (co-occurrence by chance)
4. Associative comorbidity (risk factor or causal link).

Burger H and Neeleman J. A glossary on psychiatric epidemiology. *Journal of Epidemiology and Community Health* 2007; **61**: 185–189.

17. A.   The rigorous, systematic review mentioned in the question was carried out by McGrath and colleagues. Prior to this, in 1986, the WHO published results from the International Pilot Study on Schizophrenia from seven countries; incidence of ICD 9 schizophrenia was estimated to be around 16 to 42 per 100 000 in a year. When schizophrenia was narrowly defined, this rate dropped to 7 to 14 per 100 000. McGrath *et al.* showed a fivefold difference in the incidence rates of schizophrenia across various sites in their systematic review and meta-analysis of various epidemiological studies on schizophrenia. According to this work, it is concluded that the median global incidence rate of schizophrenia is 15 per 100 000; but this global rate is not as meaningful as site-specific rates due to the degree of variation demonstrated. This view is endorsed by the AESOP study, which showed significant variation in incidence of schizophrenia among three major cities in England.

McGrath J, Saha S, Welham J *et al.* A systematic review of the incidence of schizophrenia: the distribution of rates and the influence of sex, urbanicity, migrant status and methodology. *BMC Medicine* 2004; **2**: 13.
Kirkbride JB, Fearon P, Morgan C *et al.* Heterogeneity in incidence rates of schizophrenia and other psychotic syndromes: findings from the 3-center AESOP study. *Archives of General Psychiatry* 2006; **63**: 250–258.

18. B.   The male to female difference in incidence of schizophrenia is estimated to be around 1.4: 1, with more males being diagnosed with the disease. The male excess persists even when factors such as age range and diagnostic criteria are taken into account; but interestingly this difference is not borne out when considering prevalence rates, suggesting that different factors exist in predisposing and perpetuating the illness. It may be related to males having higher mortality rates than females with schizophrenia or increased predominance of females in late-onset schizophrenia.

McGrath JJ. The surprisingly rich contours of schizophrenia epidemiology. *Archives of General Psychiatry* 2007; **64**: 14–16.

19. C.   Being born in an urban area increases the risk of schizophrenia twofold compared to individuals born in a rural area. Living in a city is also noted to increase incidence of schizophrenia. The incidence of schizophrenia is three to five times more common in migrants than a native population (median 4.6); this difference reduces to 1.8 when considering prevalence rates. Fluctuations in schizophrenia incidence have been reported over many decades. This may be related to changing structure of the population. Irrespective of broad or narrow definitions, the incidence of schizophrenia has definitely increased in certain urban areas over the last 40 years.

McGrath J, Saha S, Welham J, *et al.* A systematic review of the incidence of schizophrenia: the distribution of rates and the influence of sex, urbanicity, migrant status and methodology. *BMC Medicine* 2004; **2**: 13.

20. B.   Lifetime prevalence needs to be distinguished from lifetime morbid risk (LMR). LMR is the probability of a person developing the disorder during entire period of their life (often a specified period, defined by the life expectancy of the population studied). LMR includes the entire lifetime of a birth cohort, both past and future, and includes those deceased at the time of the survey.

Saha S, Chant D, Welham J, and McGrath J. A systematic review of the prevalence of schizophrenia. *PLoS Medicine* 2005; **2**: e141.

21. B.   For low-incidence disorders such as schizophrenia, summation of age-specific incidence rates gives approximate lifetime morbid risk values. The lifetime morbid risk for schizophrenia is 7.2/1000.

Saha S, Chant D, Welham J, and McGrath J. A systematic review of the prevalence of schizophrenia. *PLoS Medicine* 2005; **2**: e141.

22. A.   The median prevalence of schizophrenia was 4.6/1000 for point prevalence, 3.3/1000 for period prevalence, and 4.0/1000 for lifetime prevalence. There were no significant differences observed between males and females, or between urban, rural, and mixed sites with respect to the prevalence rates of schizophrenia. Migrants and homeless people had higher rates of schizophrenia and developing countries had lower prevalence rates.

Saha S, Chant D, Welham J, and McGrath J. A systematic review of the prevalence of schizophrenia. *PLoS Medicine* 2005; **2**: e141.

23. D.   The lifetime morbidity risk estimated for schizophrenia is around 7 per 1000 people in the population.

Saha S, Chant D, Welham J, and McGrath J. A systematic review of the prevalence of schizophrenia. *PLoS Medicine* 2005; **2**: e141.

24. D.   Population attributable fraction refers to the proportion of a disease in the whole population that the group exposed to specific risk factors represents. It is calculated by finding out the difference between incidence rates in the total population and the exposed population, and expressing this difference as a proportion of the total population's incidence rate. It is different from simple attributable risk, which expresses the difference in incidence rates between the exposed and non-exposed groups. Winter/ spring birth increases the risk of schizophrenia to a small extent (RR 1.11), but as the prevalence of birth itself is common in winter/ spring, 10.5% of all schizophrenia incidences can be attributed to the seasonal birth. The winter/ spring excess is positively associated with latitude.

McGrath JJ. Variations in the incidence of schizophrenia: data versus dogma. *Schizophrenia Bulletin* 2006; **32**: 195–197.

25. D.   If the measurement methodologies differ between how a case is ascertained for incidence and prevalence, then such differences will be uniformly present across various sites. Recall bias will not influence incidences measured using case notes or case registers. On the other hand, lifetime prevalence rates are susceptible to recall bias. Respondent bias, if present, must again operate uniformly and should affect various areas consistently, provided the same methods are used. A fatal disease must reduce prevalence rates uniformly. The most likely explanation is that the factors predisposing or precipitating the onset are different from the factors that serve to maintain the illness chronicity.

Saha S, Chant D, Welham J, and McGrath J. A systematic review of the prevalence of schizophrenia. *PLoS Medicine* 2005; **2**: e141.

26. A.   ESEMeD was the first major multicentre European psychiatric epidemiological study; it was not conducted in the UK. It used both Composite International Diagnostic Interview (CIDI) version 3.0 (WHO) and Structured Clinical Interview for DSM Disorders (SCID) based clinical diagnosis (DSM IV criteria). ESEMeD is a part of the World Mental Health Survey Initiative of the WHO. The results showed that 1 in 4 adults in Europe had a lifetime presence of a mental disorder and 1 in 10 had a mental disorder in the last year; 14.7% had a lifetime history of mood disorder (major depression only, 13%), while 14% had anxiety (specific phobia only, 8%), and 5.2% had a lifetime alcohol-use disorder. The highest rate of mental disorder was in the age group 18–24.

Alonso J and Lepine JP. Overview of key data from the European Study of the Epidemiology of Mental Disorders (ESEMeD). *Journal of Clinical Psychiatry* 2007; **68** (Suppl. 2): 3–9.

27. D.   Also called the filter model, the 'pathways of care' model was developed by Goldberg and Huxley to account for how mental illness interacts with the health-care system. Five levels of mental illness occurrence were described: the community, the primary-care attendees, the correctly diagnosed primary-care attendees (in whom the mental illness has been recognized), the level of the psychiatrist, and that at the level of psychiatric in-patient care. Four filters explain the decreasing incidence when going from the general population to in-patient psychiatric care:
1. At the level of the patient himself or herself (recognition)
2. At the level of the general practitioner (recognition, decision to treat, decision to refer)
3. At the out-patient level of the mental health-care system
4. At the in-patient admission level.
Occupational health resources are not major filters in this model.

Burger H and Neeleman J. A glossary on psychiatric epidemiology. *Journal of Epidemiology and Community Health* 2007; **61**: 185–189.

28. A.   Persistence is defined as the total number of patients with lifetime prevalence of a disorder who also satisfy a defined period prevalence, say 12 months, criteria at the time of survey. It is a measure of illness chronicity, response to treatment, and burden.

Burger H and Neeleman J. A glossary on psychiatric epidemiology. *Journal of Epidemiology and Community Health* 2007; **61**: 185–189.

29. B.   The Epidemiological Catchment Area study (ECA) was an investigation of the prevalence of psychiatric morbidity which was undertaken during 1976–80 in five sites in the USA. More than 20 000 people were interviewed using the Diagnostic Interview Schedule (DIS). ECA is regarded as a milestone study in psychiatric epidemiology, after which a new generation of epidemiological enquiry concentrating on community samples flourished. However, ECA was criticized for its use of lifetime diagnoses, which may be unreliable due to recollection bias. DIS was the foremost layperson-usable diagnostic instrument designed for psychiatric diagnoses.

Burger H and Neeleman J. A glossary on psychiatric epidemiology. *Journal of Epidemiology and Community Health* 2007; **61**: 185–189.

30. E.   The differential outcome of schizophrenia between developed and developing nations was first highlighted through the results of the International Pilot Study on Schizophrenia conducted by the WHO (IPSS). IPSS assessed 1202 persons diagnosed with schizophrenia in nine countries. The results showed that persons with schizophrenia in the 'developing' world (e.g. Columbia, India, and Nigeria) had better outcomes than persons in 'developed' countries (e.g. Moscow, London, Washington, Prague, and Aarhus in Denmark). In total, 52% of persons in the developing countries were assessed to be in the 'best' outcome category (defined as a single episode only, followed by full or partial recovery) compared with 39% in the developed countries. There was a claim that acute onset of psychosis, being more common in the developing nations, confounded the IPSS results, but a subsequent, large-scale, multinational study sponsored by WHO, excluded mode of onset as being a confounding factor for the observed differences in outcome. Differential follow-up rates, differential outcome measures, differential sex and age distribution, and diagnostic ambiguities did not confound the above results, as proved later by Hopper and Wanderling.

Hopper K and Wanderling J. Revisiting the developed versus developing country distinction in course and outcome in schizophrenia: results from ISoS, the WHO collaborative follow-up project. International Study of Schizophrenia. *Schizophrenia Bulletin* 2000; **26**: 835–846.

31. B. Determinants of Outcome of Severe Mental Disorder and the reduction of disability study (DOSMeD) was conducted by WHO primarily to explore the nature of the differential outcome between developed and developing nations shown by the International Pilot Study of Schizophrenia (IPSS). DOSMeD used more rigorous criteria and followed more than 1300 patients in 10 countries and, similar to the IPSS, discovered that the highest rates of recovery occurred in the developing world. The Netherlands Mental Health Survey and Incidence Study (NEMESIS study) was not a multinational study. DEPRES stands for Depression Research in European Society study. DEPRES was the first pan-European, six-country, multinational study on the prevalence of depression in the general population.

Lepine JP, Gastpar M, Mendlewicz J, and Tylee A. Depression in the community: the first pan-European study DEPRES (Depression Research in European Society). *International Clinical Psychopharmacology* 1997; **12**: 19–29.

Edgerton RB and Cohen A. Culture and schizophrenia: the DOSMD challenge. *British Journal of Psychiatry* 1994; **164**: 222–231.

32. A. The WMH Survey Consortium was formed in 1998 and 28 countries were included in a large, ambitious population survey across countries at different economical stages of development. The method employed was a multistage household probability survey. Important findings from the WMH survey initiative were:
1. Prevalence of mental disorders varies widely across countries.
2. Anxiety disorder is the most common (except Ukraine), followed by mood disorders (except Nigeria and Beijing where substance use was joint second).
3. The USA has highest prevalence rate for any disorder.
4. In all surveyed countries, severity was associated with treatment seeking. Those in developed countries obtained more treatment than those in developing nations.
5. Interestingly, a substantial proportion of non-cases were receiving treatment. This proportion was more in developed than less developed nations. This meant that most people receiving treatment are either mild cases or non-cases and not severely ill.

WHO World Mental Health Survey Consortium. Prevalence, severity, and unmet need for treatment of mental disorders in the World Health Organization World Mental Health Surveys. *JAMA* 2004; **291**: 2581–2590.

33. C. ESEMeD is the first major, multicentre, European psychiatric epidemiological study. ESEMeD is a part of World Mental health survey initiative of the WHO. Six European countries (not including the UK) were surveyed and a 60% response rate was achieved. The results showed that the highest rate of mental disorder was in the age group 18–24. Notably, while surveys such as NCS and NEMESIS excluded elderly populations, ESEMeD had nearly one in two respondents over 65 years of age.

ESEMeD/MHEDEA 2000 Investigators. Prevalence of mental disorders in Europe: results from the European Study of the Epidemiology of Mental Disorders (ESEMeD) project. *Acta Psychiatrica Scandinavia* 2004; **109** (Suppl. 420): 21–27.

34. A.   According to the ESEMeD survey, only 37% of Europeans with mood disorders and 21% with anxiety disorders sought help from health-care services. Only 21% of depressed patients received antidepressants in a year. One-third of identified cases had consulted their general practitioner in the preceding 12 months. Nearly one-third of those who sought help had never seen a mental health professional. Nearly 21% remained untreated in spite of seeking help. Comorbidity significantly influenced disability and functional impairment.

ESEMeD/MHEDEA 2000 Investigators. Prevalence of mental disorders in Europe: results from the European Study of the Epidemiology of Mental Disorders (ESEMeD) project. *Acta Psychiatrica Scandinavia* 2004; **109** (Suppl. 420): 21–27.

35. B.   Panic can exist in different forms. Major classification systems recognize panic disorder, agoraphobia, and comorbid panic disorder with agoraphobia. DSM considers panic disorder as a primary dysfunction while ICD focuses on agoraphobia. To diagnose panic disorder there must be frequent panic attacks within a specified time interval. It is increasingly realized that panic attacks can occur without fully satisfying panic disorder criteria. The National Comorbidity Survey Replication (NCS-R) collected data on four composite groups: isolated panic attacks, panic attacks with agoraphobia, panic disorder, and panic disorder with agoraphobia. Lifetime prevalence of panic attacks was only 28% compared to 4.7% who had a diagnosis of lifetime panic disorder only. Panic with agoraphobia had around 1% lifetime prevalence.

Kessler RC, Chiu WT, Jin R *et al.* The epidemiology of panic attacks, panic disorder, and agoraphobia in the National Comorbidity Survey Replication. *Archives of General Psychiatry* 2006; **63**: 415–424.

36. A.   ESEMeD revealed the degree of unmet health-care needs in Europe. A significant number of those with depression do not seek treatment. Of those depressed patients who seek help, most receive care from primary-care physicians. Only 21% of those who seek health-care support have seen a psychiatrist in the last 12 months.

Alonso J, Kovess V, Angermeyer MC *et al.* Population level of unmet need for mental healthcare in Europe. *British Journal of Psychiatry* 2007; **190**: 299–306.

37. A.   According to the National Comorbidity Survey Replication, mean age of onset of any panic attack irrespective of diagnosis is around 22 years.

Kessler RC, Chiu WT, Jin R *et al.* The epidemiology of panic attacks, panic disorder, and agoraphobia in the National Comorbidity Survey Replication. *Archives of General Psychiatry* 2006; **63**: 415–424.

38. D.   As a general rule, all anxiety disorders are more common in women than men. Notable exceptions are OCD and social phobia. OCD is more common in boys than girls, but equally common in adult men and women. Men outnumber women in seeking treatment for social phobia. It is not clear whether men suffer from a more severe form of social phobia or the level of impairment caused by social phobia is more for men than women.

Sadock BJ and Sadock VA. *Kaplan and Sadock's Synopsis of Psychiatry: Behavioral Sciences/Clinical Psychiatry*, 10th edn. Lippincott Williams and Wilkins, 2007, p. 597.

39. A. The estimated lifetime prevalence of blood–injection–injury phobia is around 3.5%. The median age of onset is around 5 to 6 years. Subjects with blood–injection–injury phobia have higher lifetime histories of fainting and seizures. Prevalence was lower in the elderly and higher in females and persons with less education. Patients with this phobia almost never seek psychiatric help, but they have significantly higher than expected lifetime prevalence of other psychiatric conditions, including substance use, depression, anxiety disorders, and OCD.

Bienvenu OJ and Eaton WW. The epidemiology of blood-injury-injection phobia. *Psychological Medicine* 1998; **28**: 1129–1136.

40. A. Reliability of diagnostic instruments used for interviews in epidemiological surveys will not change by having two independent observers, if the instrument is self-rated by the patients themselves. Similarly, descriptive responses could lower the reliability as they are prone to errors of interpretation. Having a short questionnaire and spending more than usual time on a questionnaire are not useful strategies to improve the reliability. According to psychometric principles, the reliability of an instrument could be increased, to a certain degree, if the number of questions regarding the same theme is increased. This was effectively utilized by the Stirling County Study when revising the instrument used to detect depression between 1950 and 1970.

Murphy JM, Laird NM, Monson RR *et al.* A 40-year perspective on the prevalence of depression: the Stirling County Study. *Archives of General Psychiatry* 2000; **57**: 209–215.

41. C. The Stirling County Study is one of the foremost psychiatric epidemiological studies. It was conducted on cross-sectional samples of the population living in Stirling County, Canada, in 1952, 1970, and 1992. The epidemiological data was revisited in 2000 and it showed that vernacular changes in semantic use of terms such as dysphoria could affect results of epidemiological surveys. Using the same diagnostic system (called DPAX-1) in 1952 and 1970, no increases in point prevalence of depression were noted, but when the same criteria were employed in 1992 a drop in prevalence was noted. This was due to a change in use of the term dysphoria in the studied population; this term went out of use by 1992, leading to a drop in the sensitivity of the diagnostic instrument DPAX-1. By increasing the number of questions exploring the mood state and changing the diagnostic system (to DPAX-2), similar prevalence rates were detected in 1992. Note that though the diagnostic categories changed between 1952 and 1992 this did not have a direct influence on the Stirling County Survey, which used a purpose-built instrument to measure the prevalence.

Murphy JM, Laird NM, Monson RR *et al.* A 40-year perspective on the prevalence of depression: the Stirling County Study. *Archives of General Psychiatry* 2000; **57**: 209–215.

42. C. Various studies, including NCS and its replication NCS-R, NESARC (National epidemiological Survey on Alcohol and Related Conditions) and ECA (Epidemiological Catchment Area Study), have implicated that lifetime prevalence of depression is changing. The Stirling County Study did not reveal such a significant change in rates of depression. This apparent change in prevalence could be attributed to the use of different diagnostic instruments. DIS (Diagnostic Interview Schedule), used in the ECA, and its modified improvised versions used in other studies relied on recall of lifetime prevalence. Significant recall bias is expected for a progressively older cohort who will deny or could not recall their depressive episodes. This might have resulted in a spurious effect. NCS used DSM IIIR (10.1% depression 12-month period prevalence) while its replication used DSM IV (8.7% depression prevalence), with its clinical impairment and distress criteria making it possible that less patients will be diagnosed with DSM IV. In fact, it was later shown that if DSM IV criteria were reapplied then prevalence of depression drops from 10.1% to 6.4% in the NCS 1994. In addition, NCS excluded all those above age 54 but included a 15 to 17 age group (in contrast to NCS-R), inadvertently choosing the most prevalent population that might have inflated the prevalence value. These flaws were absent in NESARC, which showed nearly doubled point prevalence estimate of depression from 3.3 to 7% from 1992 to 2002.

Hasin DS, Goodwin RD, Stinson FS *et al.* Epidemiology of major depressive disorder: Results From the National Epidemiologic Survey on Alcoholism and Related Conditions. *Archives of General Psychiatry* 2005; **62**: 1097–1106.

43. A. A nationally representative sample of nearly 8500 adults aged 16–74 years living in private households in Great Britain were interviewed by lay interviewers and were classified according to their score on the Clinical Interview Schedule–Revised (Psychiatric morbidity survey, Office of National Statistics). The Psychosis Screening questionnaire was used to collect self-reported symptoms of psychosis. In the sample, 4.2% said that there had been times when they heard or saw things that other people could not, but only 0.7% reported hearing voices saying quite a few words or sentences when there was no-one around that might account for it.

Johns LC, Singleton N, Murray RM *et al.* Prevalence and correlates of self-reported psychotic symptoms in the British population. *British Journal of Psychiatry* 2004; **185**: 298–305.

44. B. In the Office of National Statistics–Psychiatric Morbidity Survey in the UK, a self-reported instrument, called the Psychosis Screening Questionnaire, was used to detect self-reported psychotic symptoms. The questionnaire measured symptoms in five domains, namely, hallucinations, hypomania, strange experiences, paranoia, and thought insertion. Nearly half of the respondents thought that they experienced at least one hypomanic symptom when questioned, but, when explored further, more than half of the respondents had valid reasons for feeling very happy for many days without a break. Only 0.6% reported their friends or relatives commenting on such a prolonged 'happy' state.

Johns LC, Singleton N, Murray RM *et al.* Prevalence and correlates of self-reported psychotic symptoms in the British population. *British Journal of Psychiatry* 2004; **185**: 298–305.

45. C. Surveys of preschool children have recorded a high prevalence of problem behaviours. The most commonly reported problem is that of bedwetting, seen in around 37% of a sample. Boys and girls show equal prevalence of these problems while those with expressive language disorders show more behavioural difficulties. Maternal depression and family discord at 3 years strongly predict behavioural disorder by the age of 8.

Richman N, Stevenson J, and Graham P. Prevalence of behaviour problems in 3 year old children: An epidemiological study in a London borough. *Journal of Child Psychology and Psychiatry* 1975; **16**: 277–287.

46. A. The Isle of Wight Study was one of the earliest epidemiological studies on children, carried out by Rutter *et al.* in 1960. In this study, all 10- to 11-year-old children in the Isle of Wight were surveyed using both parent and teacher questionnaires separately. A 5.7% prevalence of diagnosable psychiatric disorders was identified. Boys had more problems than girls in the ratio 2: 1. But only 10% of these children were known to psychiatric services at the time of this study.

Rutter M, Tizand J, Yule W *et al.* Research report: Isle of Wight Studies, 1964–1974. *Psychological Medicine* 1976; **6**: 313–332.

47. B. It is observed that adolescents have more psychiatric difficulties than younger children. The Isle of Wight Study was repeated when the cohort was around 14–15 years of age and the prevalence of psychiatric disorders was found to have increased from 5.7% to 8%. Marital disharmony predicted development of psychiatric problems by adolescence. A similar study carried out using a cohort followed up at Dunedin, New Zealand, revealed similar results.

Graham P and Rutter M. Psychiatric disorder in the young adolescent. *Proceedings of the Royal Society of Medicine* 1973; **66**: 1226–1229.

McGee R, Feehan M, Williams S *et al.* DSM-III disorders in a large sample of adolescents. *Journal of the American Academy of Child and Adolescent Psychiatry* 1990; **29**: 611–619.

48. E. In most of the large-scale epidemiological surveys of the last two decades, screening is carried out in a population sample using layperson-administered, structured tools to identify 'caseness'. This is later followed by clinician-led diagnostic assessment to confirm such cases. It has been shown repeatedly that layperson diagnostic instruments diagnose more mental illness than those identified by clinician administered, standardized instruments. The agreement between these two types of diagnostic tools is poor, around a kappa of 0.1 to 0.4 only, but no single instrument can be claimed to be superior for case ascertainment purposes.

Brugha T, Bebbington PE, Jenkins R *et al.* Cross validation of a general population survey diagnostic interview: a comparison of CIS-R with SCAN ICD-10 diagnostic categories. *Psychological Medicine* 1999; **5**: 1029–1042.

49. D. Using the data from 17 countries that participated in the WMH survey initiative, the cross-national lifetime prevalence of suicidal ideation is estimated to be 9.2%. Planning for suicide is estimated to occur in 3.1% while actual attempts take place in 2.7% of the sample; 60% of transitions from ideation to plan and attempt occur within the first year after ideation onset. Consistent, cross-national risk factors included being female, younger, less educated, unmarried, and having a mental disorder.

Nock MK, Borges G, Bromet EJ *et al.* Cross-national prevalence and risk factors for suicidal ideation, plans and attempts. *British Journal of Psychiatry* 2008; **192**: 98–105.

50. D. The significant risk factors strongly related to suicidal ideation in cross-sectional samples are being female, previously married, age less than 25 years, being poorly educated, and having one or more diagnosable psychiatric disorders. These risk factors are strongly associated with suicidal ideation rather than conversion of ideas to attempts. In fact, suicides are more common in men than women across all age groups.

Nock MK, Borges G, Bromet EJ et al. Cross-national prevalence and risk factors for suicidal ideation, plans and attempts. *British Journal of Psychiatry* 2008; **192**: 98–105.

51. C. The term incidence density refers to the number of new cases observed in a defined period in a population per person-year of observation.

Sadock BJ and Sadock VA. *Kaplan and Sadock's Comprehensive Textbook of Psychiatry*, 8th edn. Lippincott Williams and Wilkins, 2004, p. 660.

52. B. To describe the development of psychiatric epidemiology, three 'generations' of studies are distinguished. Around 16 psychiatric epidemiological studies, carried out before World War II, belong to the first generation. These studies focused primarily on the health-care agency-registered prevalence of mental disorders in relation to community characteristics. The second generation of psychiatric epidemiological studies followed an increased interest in the diagnostic criteria, classification, and nomenclature of psychiatric disorders after World War II, when nearly 60 studies appeared. These were mainly field surveys, conducted in unstructured clinical interviews. Consequently, the reliability of these studies was low. The third-generation studies started around 1970, with more effort put into increasing the reliability of psychiatric diagnoses. A major objective of the third-generation studies is to obtain precise estimates of prevalence and incidence of specific mental disorders, whereas second-generation studies focused on mental ill-health in general. It is claimed that a fourth generation of psychiatric epidemiological studies is in the making. This includes studies that include comprehensive sets of biological markers such as brain imaging, cerebrospinal fluid examinations, blood sampling, etc. in the large-scale, cross-sectional surveys.

Burger H and Neeleman J. A glossary on psychiatric epidemiology. *Journal of Epidemiology and Community Health* 2007; **61**: 185–189.
Skoog I. Psychiatric epidemiology of old age: the H70 study—NAPE lecture 2003. *Acta Psychiatrica Scandinavica* 2004: **109**: 4–18.

53. D. Using the Camberwell Assessment of Needs Schedule, Bebbington et al. determined the unmet need for psychiatric care to be around 10% of the sample assessed from inner south London. Less than half of all potentially achievable needs were met in this sample. There was only partial overlap between diagnosis and an adjudged need for treatment, that is there was a significant section of the sample that had a need for treatment irrespective of diagnostic categorization. It was concluded that most of these needs could be met at the primary care level.

Bebbington PE, Marsden L, and Brewin CR. The need for psychiatric treatment in the general population: The Camberwell needs for care Survey. *Psychological Medicine* 1997; **27**: 821–834.

54. A. As a part of the WMH Survey Initiative, adult respondents were screened for criteria of ADHD in a cross-national sample. The estimates of ADHD prevalence averaged 3.4%, with lower prevalence in lower income countries (1.9%) compared with higher-income countries (4.2%). A high degree of comorbidity was noted for adult ADHD, and, interestingly, in most low-income countries the comorbidities were treated more than the ADHD itself. The treatment for adult ADHD was better in developed countries.

Fayyad J, De Graaf R, Kessler RC et al. Cross-national prevalence and correlates of adult attention-deficit hyperactivity disorder. *British Journal of Psychiatry* 2007; **190**: 402–409.

55. D. 'Years of potential life lost' (YPLL) is a measure of the impact of premature mortality on a population. It is calculated as the sum of the differences between some predetermined end point (commonly the life expectancy of population or age 65 as standard) and the ages of death for those who died before that end point. Crude mortality is not specific for age distribution of mortality. The infant mortality rate does not pick up deaths occurring after 1 year of age.

US Department of Health and Human Services. *Principles of Epidemiology*, 2nd edn. www2a.cdc. gov/phtn/catalog/pdf-file/Epi_Course.pdf (accessed 19.08.2008), p. 112.

56. D. AESOP (Aetiology and Ethnicity study of Schizophrenia and other Psychoses) was a UK-based study on the incidence of psychosis in three major cities—London, Nottingham, and Bristol. AESOP explored ethnicity differences in the incidence of psychosis in these cities and found that all psychoses were more common in the black and minority ethnic group, with an incidence rate ratio of 3.6. When adjusted statistically for confounding factors, this reduced to an adjusted incidence rate ratio of 2.9. It was also noted that the incidence of all psychoses was higher in south-east London than Bristol or Nottingham. The UK700 study explored the differences in outcome between various types of service delivery, that is community teams and assertive outreach models. The PRISM psychosis study analysed the effect of setting up community treatment teams on various outcomes and satisfaction measures for service users.

Morgan C, Dazzan P, Morgan K *et al*. First episode psychosis and ethnicity: initial findings from the AESOP study. *World Psychiatry* 2006; **5**: 40–46.

57. E. Lifespan surveys across elderly population are limited. The H70 study refers to a meticulous, large–scale, longitudinal data collection from individuals over age 70 (born 1901–1902, observations started in 1971) in Sweden. It included detailed examinations of ageing and age-related somatic and psychiatric disorders, such as physical examinations performed by geriatricians, electrocardiograms, chest X-rays, a battery of blood tests, nutritional factors, anthropometric measurements, psychosocial background factors, and psychometric tests performed by psychologists. It has provided a rich source of data on elderly populations in Europe. The psychiatric data available from the H70 show that approximately 30% of those older than 75 years have mental disorders of some form.

Skoog I. Psychiatric epidemiology of old age: the H70 study—NAPE lecture 2003. *Acta Psychiatrica Scandinavica* 2004: **109**: 4–18.

58. C. EURO-DEP is a European consortium to study the epidemiology of depression in later life. This utilizes a secondary research method wherein existing datasets on epidemiology in late-life depression are pooled and a new instrument, called EURO-D, to diagnose depression using the various heterogeneous scales from these studies has been devised. The EURO-D scale was developed from 12 items of the Geriatric Mental State and validated against other scales and expert diagnosis. Meta-analysis of nearly 14 000 subjects interviewed in various studies using the Geriatric Mental State, yielded a mean level of depression of 12.3%; the prevalence in women was 14.1% and men 8.6%. DEPRES (Depression Research in European Society) is the first large, pan-European survey of depression in the community. It is not secondary research. The Netherlands Mental Health Survey and Incidence Study (NEMESIS) is a prospective study of the prevalence, incidence, and course of psychiatric disorders in a sample of Dutch adults aged 18 to 64.

Copeland JRM, Beekman ATF, Braam AW *et al*. Depression among older people in Europe: the EURODEP studies *World Psychiatry* 2004; **3**: 45–49.

59. E.   Postpartum depression has no specific causal factors. Though numerous risk factors, such as social isolation and adverse life events, are associated with the incidence of postnatal depression, none of these factors are specific enough to differentiate postnatal depression from depression occurring during other phases of a woman's life. Depression is common in perimenopausal, peripubertal, and child-rearing or pregnant women. Postpartum depression is essentially same disease as major depression occurring at other times, with respect to its classificatory status. Postpartum depression is not a continuum of postpartum psychosis, which is more closely associated with bipolar illness. The Edinburgh Postnatal Depression Scale is a self-rated scale with 10 items. It is a screening tool for detecting depression in mothers. Postpartum psychosis occurs following around 1 per 1000 live births. The recurrence rate of postpartum psychosis is about 1 in 4 subsequent pregnancies.

Brockington P. Post partum psychiatric disorders. *Lancet* 2004; **363**: 303–310.

60. E.   Suicide rates in male mental health-service users are always higher than female service users irrespective of the age group. The male: female suicide rate is around 3: 1. The gender difference is most pronounced at age 25 to 34, where nearly 80% are males. The divide is less steep in those more than 75 years of age where nearly 60% are males.

Swinson N, Ashim B, Windfuhr K *et al.* National confidential inquiry into suicide and homicide by people with mental illness: new directions. *Psychiatric Bulletin* 2007; **31**: 161–163.

61. A.   Sensitivity of a diagnostic test refers to the proportion of diseased subjects who have a positive test result (true positive rate). If it is 80%, then out of 10 truly diseased (anxious) people, eight will be correctly identified using the instrument. Specificity refers to the proportion of the non-diseased subjects who have a negative test result (true negative rate). So nine out of 10 people without anxiety will be correctly identified as 'normal' using the instrument. Choices D and E refer to positive and negative predictive values, respectively. Positive predictive value refers to the proportion of test-positive subjects who are actually diseased. For the given values of sensitivity and specificity this is 8/9. Negative predictive value refers to the proportion of test-negative subjects who are in fact 'normal'. For the given values of sensitivity and specificity this is 2/11.

Lawrie SM, McIntosh AM, and Rao S. *Critical Appraisal for Psychiatry.* Churchill Livingstone, 2000, p. 96.

62. B.   A receiver–operator curve is used to decide the optimal cut-off of a screening test. A funnel plot is used in systematic reviews and meta-analyses to demonstrate publication bias. The likelihood ratio of a negative result in diagnostic evaluation is given by a likelihood nomogram. The survival rates of inception cohorts in a follow-up study are demonstrated using a Kaplan–Meier curve. Kappa statistics can be used to test inter-rater reliability of a new instrument.

Lawrie SM, McIntosh AM, and Rao S. *Critical Appraisal for Psychiatry.* Churchill Livingstone, 2000, p. 146.

63. B.   Cohort studies can be differentiated from case–control studies on the basis of the time of exposure and duration of observation. In case–control studies the exposure has occurred in the past, unknown to the researcher. Cases and controls are independently recruited and differential exposure is ascertained in the two groups. In cohort studies, recruitment into a study takes place as soon as or as and when the exposure occurs (exposure cohort). In this question, exposure is the traumatic flight. Outcome is prospectively observed development of PTSD. Therefore this is a cohort study.

Lawrie SM, McIntosh AM, and Rao S. *Critical Appraisal for Psychiatry.* Churchill Livingstone, 2000, p. 30.

64. A. Inception cohort refers to all individuals assembled at a given point based on some factor, for example common demography or common life experience. In the above example, following a survey, a group of individuals with similar experience of auditory hallucinations are followed up prospectively. Hence they constitute an inception cohort. Open cohort refers to recruiting the cohort over an extended period of time instead of choosing the same point in time. In most open cohorts the individual subjects are followed up for variable time intervals until the study is completed.

Laupacis A, Wells G, Richardson WS, and Tugwell P. Users' guides to the medical literature. V. How to use an article about prognosis. *JAMA* 1994; **271**: 234–237.

65. D. Widely known as the Bradford Hill's criteria for causal association, demonstration of the following helps to ascertain cause–effect relationships:
1. Temporal association: The cause X must have occurred before the effect (disease) Y.
2. Dose–response relationship: the higher the X, the more the Y.
3. Consistency of association: whenever Y is present X is present and vice versa.
4. Strength of association must be high.
5. Biological plausibility: X has a biologically sensible causal pathway leading to Y.
6. Specificity: X is associated with Y only, not a wide range of other diseases.
7. There must be experimental evidence to support the claims.

Holt RIG and Peveler RC. Antipsychotic drugs and diabetes—an application of the Austin Bradford Hill criteria. *Diabetologia* 2006; **49**: 1467–1476.

66. E. Cross-sectional surveys are best suited for calculating epidemiological measures such as prevalence rates. To detect incidence rates the cross-sectional survey must be conducted at two different time points (to ascertain 'new' cases). To detect point prevalence rates a single cross-sectional study should be sufficient.

Lawrie SM, McIntosh AM, and Rao S. *Critical Appraisal for Psychiatry*. Churchill Livingstone, 2000, p. 23.

67. B. Studies show that exposure to maternal drinking in adolescence is a strong risk factor for the development of alcohol problems in early adulthood. For males and females, no association was found between either birth factors or childhood factors and a lifetime diagnosis of alcohol disorders at age 21 years. Externalizing symptoms and maternal factors at age 14 years were significantly associated with alcohol problems. For youths aged 14 years, maternal moderate alcohol consumption accounted for the highest percentage of attributable risk among those exposed.

Alati R, Najman JM, Kinner SA *et al*. Early predictors of adult drinking: a birth cohort study. *American Journal of Epidemiology* 2005; **162**: 1098–1107.

68. C. Accuracy refers to the extent to which results are close to the truth. In psychometry, it is used interchangeably (and controversially) with the term validity. Precision refers to the extent to which results are consistent or close to each other and hence are reproducible. The new test produces results that are close to the truth as observed from the gold standard results. Hence it is accurate, but the magnitude of measured outcome varies widely among the tested population. Hence it is not precise.

Streiner DL and Norman GR. "Precision" and "accuracy": two terms that are neither. *Journal of Clinical Epidemiology* 2006; **59**: 327–330.

69. C.   Though OCD was previously thought to be quite rare, recent evidence suggests this is not the case. A lifetime prevalence rate of 2–3% has been suggested. OCD is among the top 20 causes of illness-related disability for people between the ages of 15 and 44. The age of onset of OCD is usually mid-to-late twenties. The female to male ratio is said to be more or less equal, though some studies suggest an excess in females. The mean age of onset for men is around 22 years, for women this is slightly delayed—around 26 years. The illness tends to be secret in most patients with a delay of several years before treatment is sought. OCD is the fourth most common mental illness in world. The disorder presents with comparable prevalence rates across various countries, with some cultural specificity to the content of obsessions.

Weissman MM, Bland RC, Canino GJ *et al*. The cross national epidemiology of obsessive compulsive disorder. The Cross National Collaborative Group. *Journal of Clinical Psychiatry* 1994; **55**: 5–10.

70. A.   The prevalence of diabetes is higher in not only schizophrenia but also in patients with bipolar I disorder (26%) and schizoaffective disorder (50%), independent of psychotropic drug use. Genetic factors have a key role in the association between schizophrenia and diabetes; up to 50% of individuals with schizophrenia were found to have a family history of type 2 diabetes in a study. The increased risk is demonstrated regardless of antipsychotic medication use. Due to frequent screening and blood test in the treatment-resistant group, the detection of hidden impaired glucose tolerance may be higher. Diabetes is estimated to be at least two to four times more prevalent in schizophrenia than in the general population, but significant variability is noted in the actual prevalence rates reported. Difficulties in developing a wide-reaching screening programme may be a source of this variability.

Bushe C and Holt R. Prevalence of diabetes and impaired glucose tolerance in patients with schizophrenia. *British Journal of Psychiatry* 2004; **184**: 67–71.

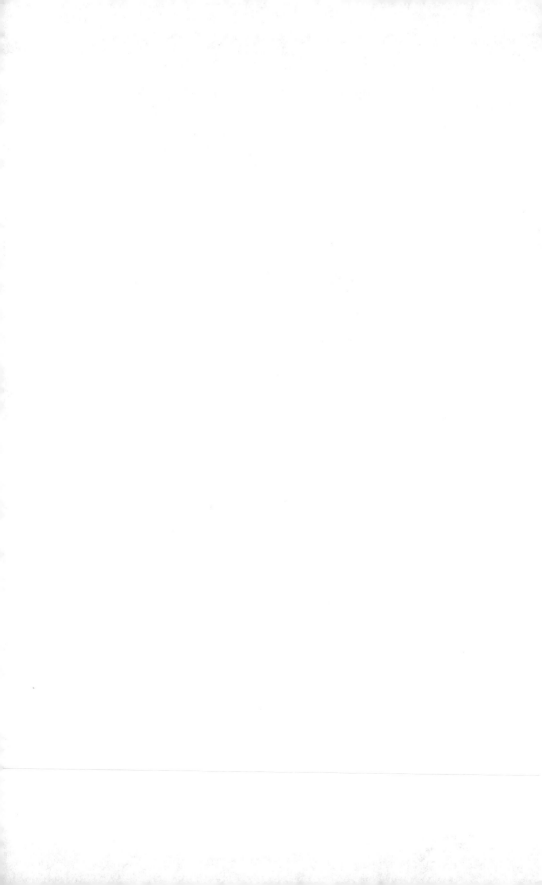

1. While measuring attitudes to abortion, the subjects are given a set of statements carefully chosen by a panel of judges beforehand. Each statement carries a pre-assigned value. The subjects are asked to indicate whether they agree or not with each statement. Which of the following methods is being used in this study?

   A. Likert Scale
   B. Osgood's Semantic Differential Scale
   C. Thurstone Scale
   D. Sociogram
   E. Scalogram

2. A boring task is administered to two groups of people. One group is paid £20 and the other is paid £1 for undertaking the task. Which of the following results is possible after completion of the task?

   A. Only the £1 group will appreciate the usefulness of the task.
   B. Only the £20 group will appreciate the usefulness of the task.
   C. Both groups will equally appreciate the task.
   D. Both groups will equally detest the task.
   E. The outcome will depend on the length of the task.

3. Measured attitudes often differ from observed behaviours. Which of the following could improve the correlation between a measured attitude and actual behaviour?

   A. Repeated measurement of attitudes
   B. Measuring attitude in a general context without hypothetical constraints
   C. Measuring the single most predictive attitude for a given behaviour
   D. Measuring attitudes with specified target, context, and time elements
   E. Postal survey of attitudes

4. A politician is trying to persuade his working-class audience to vote in favour of his space science policy. Which of the following will produce a successful persuasion?
    A. Being highly credible with respect to the policy
    B. Appearing strikingly different from the audience
    C. Providing an overview of both good and bad aspects of his policy
    D. Inducing a high degree of fear regarding the consequences of non-acceptance
    E. Introducing the topic by emphasizing that the policy has been made by a panel unknown to the politician

5. Which of the following statements is incorrect with respect to the role of fear in changing one's attitudes?
    A. Absence of fear can inhibit attitude change
    B. Extreme fear can inhibit attitude change
    C. In the presence of precise instructions, fear facilitates attitude change
    D. Feeling of vulnerability decreases attitude change
    E. Fear and attitude change are related by an inverted U shaped curve

6. An autistic child is successively reinforced for behaviours ranging from making eye contact, attending to therapist's speech, and imitating speech sounds until sentences are uttered in normal social contexts. This technique is called
    A. Shaping
    B. Chaining
    C. Flooding
    D. Aversion therapy
    E. Token economy

7. A smoker is made aware of numerous health problems that could occur due to smoking. If the smoker attempts to reduce the dissonance between his smoking behaviour and health beliefs, which of the following is least likely to happen?
    A. Change in smoking behaviour
    B. Removing the dissonant health belief
    C. Minimizing the importance of one's health
    D. Adding a new belief, for example 'filter cigarettes are safe'
    E. Denying the strength of evidence for smoking-related harm

8. Inducing cognitive dissonance is an important therapeutic approach in which of the following treatments?
    A. Systematic desensitization
    B. Token therapy
    C. Interpersonal therapy
    D. Motivation enhancement therapy
    E. Brief psychodynamic therapy

9. Which of the following terms describes an evaluative rather than a descriptive stand one holds about oneself?

   A. Self-image
   B. Bodily self
   C. Self-esteem
   D. Self-consciousness
   E. Ideal self

10. Behavioural couples therapy is a treatment approach used in which of the following conditions?

   A. Alcohol use disorder
   B. Premature ejaculation
   C. Sex offender therapy
   D. Delusional jealousy
   E. Dependent personality disorder

11. Which of the following factors plays a role in the development of self-concept?

   A. Reaction of others towards oneself
   B. Social comparison one makes with others
   C. Social roles one plays in everyday life
   D. Identification with a social group
   E. All of the above

12. In a prosperous country with good tolerance, a famine strikes all of a sudden. This is followed by a surge of intolerance between two racial tribes wherein the minorities are discriminated against. Which of the following theories can explain this prejudice?

   A. Relative deprivation theory
   B. Group membership theory
   C. Social identity theory
   D. Authoritarian personality theory
   E. Cognitive dissonance theory

13. The term 'nomothetic' in personality theories refers to which of the following concepts?

   A. Personality is unique for each individual
   B. Individuals have overlapping personality traits
   C. Ambiguity can induce personality variables to come to the surface
   D. Personality is influenced by pathological processes
   E. Personality is not measurable but can only be described

14. **Which of the following distinctions between prejudice and discrimination holds true?**
    A. Prejudice is a behaviour while discrimination is an attitude
    B. Discrimination and prejudice are both attitudes
    C. Prejudice is an attitude while discrimination is a behaviour
    D. Discrimination has both cognitive and behavioural components
    E. Prejudice can only be negative while discrimination could be positive or negative

15. **Which of the following is the average age by which the concept of theory of mind becomes established in children?**
    A. 2 to 2 1/2 years
    B. 1 to 1 1/2 years
    C. 3 1/2 to 4 years
    D. 6 to 7 years
    E. 8 to 9 years

16. **Which of the following is often the first social category learnt by a developing child?**
    A. Concept of individualism
    B. Gender concept
    C. Race concept
    D. Religion concept
    E. Age concept

17. **The average age by which most humans develop self-recognition is**
    A. 1 to 3 months
    B. 16 to 18 months
    C. 18 to 20 months
    D. 12 to 14 months
    E. 4 to 6 months

18. **'Touching the dot' is a popular psychological experiment to demonstrate which of the following concepts?**
    A. Self-esteem
    B. Gestalt theory of perception
    C. Self-recognition
    D. Visual perception
    E. Depth perception

19. **After her failure in an examination in spite of hard work, a candidate starts regarding the failure as a stepping stone to success. Which of the following explains such an attitude?**
    A. Effort justification dissonance
    B. Denial mechanism
    C. Passive–aggressive personality
    D. Narcissistic personality
    E. Learned helplessness

20. **Which of the following methods of measuring attitudes uses bipolar adjectives?**

    A. Likert scale
    B. Osgood's Semantic Differential scale
    C. Thurstone Scale
    D. Sociogram
    E. Scalogram

21. **While undergoing couples therapy, each partner agrees a way of rewarding the other when the desired behaviour is carried out. This is called**

    A. Sculpting
    B. Role reversal
    C. Socratic questioning
    D. Guided discovery
    E. Reciprocity negotiation

22. **The id impulses are counterbalanced by defence mechanisms mediated by ego. When id retaliates against the moral imposed by superego, which of the following results?**

    A. Repressions
    B. Obsessions
    C. Suppression
    D. Repetition compulsion
    E. Dissociation

23. **A 45-year-old depressed man becomes clingy and tearful when his wife visits him. He adapts a fetal posture and sleeps on her lap. Which of the following is being exhibited?**

    A. Repression
    B. Sadism
    C. Retardation
    D. Regression
    E. Degeneration

24. **According to psychoanalytic theories of anxiety which of the following anxieties is the most primitive in development?**

    A. Disintegration anxiety
    B. Superego anxiety
    C. Castration anxiety
    D. Separation anxiety
    E. Stranger anxiety

25. **Which of the following applies to Jungian modification of psychoanalysis?**
    A. Active imagination is encouraged
    B. Thanatos or death instinct forms the dominant concept
    C. Uninterrupted, lifelong psychotherapy is encouraged
    D. Jungian therapy is based on object relations theory
    E. Play therapy is encouraged

26. **A psychiatric trainee is reprimanded for using social network websites with explicit sexual content while at work. He explains that such breaks are very important while doing a stressful job and preventing web access at work will only make him less efficient at work. Which of the following defence mechanisms is he using?**
    A. Intellectualization
    B. Reaction formation
    C. Projection
    D. Rationalization
    E. Sublimation

27. **The term cathexis in psychoanalysis refers to which of the following?**
    A. The junction between two neurones
    B. Re-enactment of childhood conflicts during a therapy session
    C. Narrating negative experiences in life without inhibition
    D. The instinctual energy stored in neurones
    E. A defence mechanism thought to act during sleep

28. **A patient attending psychotherapy sessions for pervasive anxiety and depression shows reduced interest in the therapy gradually, after the first eight sessions. When questioned she replies that she continues to attend only to achieve the satisfaction of 'being looked-after'. Which of the following processes explains the above?**
    A. Counter transference
    B. Transference neurosis
    C. Transference regression
    D. Aggression turned outwards
    E. Narcissistic transference

29. **Which of the following themes is central to Kleinian psychoanalysis?**
    A. Relationship between past and present life
    B. Relationship between libidinal desires and routine events
    C. Relationship between internal and external world
    D. Relationship between collective and individual unconscious
    E. Relationship between ideal and real self

30. **Which of the following is true according to the social identity theory?**
    A. Individuals often choose between social identity and personal identity
    B. Each individual has a single specific social identity
    C. In-group attitudes help preserve social identity
    D. Social identity cannot influence self-esteem directly
    E. Discriminatory behaviour is not related to one's social identity

31. **In a therapy group for patients with emotional instability, a 34-year-old lady realizes how her interactions differ significantly in the group compared to her past relationships. Which of the following processes is described in this scenario?**
    A. Positive group identification
    B. Group cohesion
    C. Corrective emotional experience
    D. Mirroring
    E. Catharsis

32. **Which of the following factors is not considered influential in achieving personal growth and change while undergoing a group therapy?**
    A. Instillation of hope
    B. Imparting information
    C. Imitative behaviour
    D. Stable administration
    E. Socialization in the group

33. **In therapeutic dramatization (psychodrama) the term protagonist refers to which of the following?**
    A. The person most loved by the patient
    B. The therapist
    C. A fellow patient who aids in treatment
    D. The patient
    E. The person most hated by the patient

34. **According to Freud's structural model of mind, which of the following is correctly arranged in order of development?**
    A. Ego, id, superego
    B. Id, ego, superego
    C. Superego, ego, id
    D. Superego, id, ego
    E. Id, superego, ego

35. **Which of the following psychosexual phases and developmental fears is correctly matched?**

    A. Oral phase: fear of annihilation
    B. Anal phase: fear of loss of loved object
    C. Genital phase: castration anxiety
    D. Latent phase: feelings of guilt
    E. Oedipal phase: fear of annihilation

36. **A therapist encourages her patient to continue avoiding the phobic object, in order to create an insight about the problems associated with such behaviour. Which of the following techniques is she using?**

    A. Triangulation
    B. Negative transference
    C. Paradoxical injunction
    D. Reframing
    E. Covert sensitization

37. **Which of the following groups has a high level of leadership activity with highly specific therapy goals?**

    A. Psychodrama
    B. Interpersonal therapy
    C. Problem-solving therapy
    D. Problem-drinkers groups
    E. Systems-centred groups

38. **Which of the following disorders and defence mechanisms is correctly paired?**

    A. Anankastic personality: projective identification
    B. Schizoid personality: splitting
    C. Conversion disorder: suppression
    D. OCD: undoing
    E. Anorexia: anticipation

39. **Which of the following is not a major principle of a therapeutic community?**

    A. Communalism
    B. Democratization
    C. Permissiveness
    D. Instillation of hope
    E. Reality confrontation

40. **Which of the following can reduce prejudice against a minority group?**

    A. Negotiating under conditions imposed by the minorities
    B. Improving social contact between members of equal status
    C. Increasing personal friendships between opposite group members
    D. Careful prevention of self-experience of prejudice by the members of dominant group
    E. Setting up competitive targets between the two groups

41. Which of the following concepts refers to the ability of an analyst to deal with repeated primitive transferences which evolve during psychotherapy without retaliation or abandonment of the patient?

A. Containing
B. Holding
C. Probing
D. Withstanding
E. Working through

42. Which of the following stages of change is most suitable to start acamprosate?

A. Precontemplation
B. Contemplation
C. Maintenance
D. Action
E. Relapse

43. When asked to recall the attachment experience in childhood, a subject gives an unelaborated account, minimizing problems faced as a child. Which of the following attachment style has this subject most likely had as a child?

A. Secure autonomous pattern
B. Insecure avoidant pattern
C. Insecure disorganized pattern
D. Insecure ambivalent pattern
E. Multiple attachment pattern

44. Deficits, disputes, and role transitions are identified in which of the following psychotherapies?

A. Dialectic behavioural therapy
B. Rational emotive therapy
C. Interpersonal therapy
D. Brief dynamic therapy
E. Motivational enhancement therapy

45. Which of the following therapies uses the terms 'snags', 'dilemmas', and 'role repertoires'?

A. Dialectic behavioural therapy
B. Rational emotive therapy
C. Interpersonal therapy
D. Cognitive analytical therapy
E. Motivational enhancement therapy

46. **Which of the following treatments was specifically developed to reduce intentional self-harm behaviour?**

    A. Dialectic behavioural therapy
    B. Rational emotive therapy
    C. Interpersonal therapy
    D. Cognitive analytical therapy
    E. Motivational enhancement therapy

47. **Your pet dog barks at your new friend who visits you at home. When you hug your friend during every subsequent visit, the dog gradually stops barking. Which of the following best explains this phenomenon?**

    A. Reciprocal determinism
    B. Reciprocal inhibition
    C. Applied relaxation
    D. Biofeedback
    E. Vicarious learning

48. **A teacher notices that one of her pupils is sleeping during her lecture while the rest are actively listening. She concludes that her lecture is boring and worthless. Which of the following cognitive distortions best suits the above description?**

    A. Arbitrary inference
    B. Catastrophic interpretation
    C. Overgeneralization
    D. Selective abstraction
    E. Dichotomous thinking

49. **Production of repetitive phonemes seen in a growing child is called babbling. Which of the following is true with respect to babbling?**

    A. Deaf–mute children do not babble.
    B. Babbling is seen around 6 weeks of age.
    C. The age of attaining the ability to babble depends on the mother tongue.
    D. Babbling takes place irrespective of the presence of adults in the vicinity.
    E. Babbling stops when the first word is learnt.

50. **In Cattell's personality theory, the 16 measured personality factors (16PF) can be termed**

    A. Surface traits
    B. Secondary traits
    C. Source traits
    D. Central traits
    E. Cardinal traits

51. While making a moral judgement on a narrated story, a girl expresses that there is no wrong in doing things which will get her candies. Which phase of moral development is she in?

    A. Universal ethical orientation
    B. Social contract orientation
    C. Conventional morality
    D. Obedience orientation
    E. Reward orientation

52. During psychotherapy, a patient starts becoming unwell after a prolonged period of good recovery, in spite of having many more sessions to come in the future. Which of the following can explain the above?

    A. Negative therapeutic reaction
    B. Termination reaction
    C. Negative transference reaction
    D. Uncovering repressed memories
    E. Resistance to change

53. Which of the following is not a cognitive variable crucial for social learning?

    A. Attention
    B. Imitative reproduction
    C. Memory retention
    D. Motivation
    E. Problem solving

54. Which of the following best describes supportive psychotherapy?

    A. It is a goal-directed psychotherapy
    B. Its primary aim is to help patients strengthen their ego defences
    C. It is generally a brief and time-limited therapy
    D. Its primary aim is to provide generic social skills training
    E. Explicit reassurance must not be given when sought by the patient

55. Which of the following cognitive distortions is characteristically seen in patients with panic attacks?

    A. Catastrophic thinking
    B. Minimization
    C. Dichotomous thinking
    D. Rationalization
    E. Overgeneralization

56. **In Milgram's obedience experiments, which of the following decreased the tendency of the subject to administer shock to a victim?**
    A. Prominent authority of experimenter
    B. Proximity of victim to the subject
    C. Proximity of the experimenter to the subject
    D. Administration of shock using a proxy or helper
    E. Removing responsibility from the subject

57. **Discussing a controversial decision in a group strengthens average individual inclinations to vote against the risky decision. What is the name given to the above process?**
    A. Obedience
    B. Conformity
    C. Groupthink
    D. Group polarization
    E. Risky shift

58. **Which of the following statements with respect to language development is incorrect?**
    A. The earliest learnt words are context bound
    B. 'Holophrases' are one-word substitutes for a whole sentence
    C. Vocabulary of word-production exceeds word-comprehension by 18 months of age
    D. Propositions are learnt later than verbs
    E. Telegraphic speech is seen after 18 months of age

59. **In a behavioural therapy session for repetitive hair pulling, the patient is asked to wear gloves when he finds himself in a stressful situation that can promote hair pulling. This technique could be termed**
    A. Self-monitoring
    B. Stimulus control
    C. Chaining
    D. Negative practice
    E. Exposure and response prevention

60. **Repeated eye movement during a conscious recollection is used as a psychotherapeutic technique in which of the following disorders?**
    A. Panic disorder
    B. Agoraphobia
    C. Compulsive skin picking
    D. PTSD
    E. Depression

61. **Which of the following is true regarding the Parental Bonding Instrument?**

- A. It is an observer-rated scale to be administered by trained child psychologists
- B. It is prone to recall bias
- C. It is used to elicit attachment style from breast feeding mothers
- D. It is used to interview school-aged children on the quality of bonding
- E. The questions are semistructured

62. **The five-areas approach to CBT includes focusing on all of the following domains of a patient's experience except**

- A. Behaviours
- B. Physical symptoms
- C. Relationships
- D. Thinking
- E. Traumatic past

63. **While administering CBT, all of the following are appropriate therapeutic processes that can be employed by a therapist except**

- A. Encouraging reduction in working hours to reduce stress
- B. Exploring the patient's illness model
- C. Setting goals and targets initially
- D. Setting tasks to be completed as homework
- E. Using the patient's own descriptive terms

64. **Which of the following is true with respect to psychoanalytic theory of depression?**

- A. Awareness of a painful thought is important for the origin of depression
- B. Anger can present as depression
- C. The concept of 'object' always refers to a parent
- D. The main source of depression is dream content
- E. Depression cannot be treated after early adulthood

65. **Which one among the following processes seen in group therapy is not associated with Wilfred Bion?**

- A. Basic assumptions
- B. Amplification
- C. Fight–flight
- D. Pairing
- E. Dependency

66. Richard is a student in sociology at the University. He favours behaviour such as reading, meditating, creative writing, and composing music, compared to his flat mate, Martin, who prefers to spend most of his time with his circle of friends. According to Jung's type trait theory of personality, Richard would best be described as an

    A. Ambivert
    B. Ectomorph
    C. Endomorph
    D. Extrovert
    E. Introvert

67. Jim is an 80-year-old man who leads a retired life with his wife Sarah. He had been a postman till he retired at the age of 60. He raised two children who are successful engineers and have families of their own. Looking back at his life, he gets a sense of fulfilment and feels that he can face approaching death with a sense of acceptance. According to Erikson, what trait does he have?

    A. Generativity
    B. Identity
    C. Integrity
    D. Isolation
    E. Self-actualization

68. Non-directiveness, unconditional positive regard, active listening, and empathy are features of a psychotherapeutic technique originated by Carl Rogers. Which of the following therapies do these terms represent?

    A. Behaviour therapy
    B. Client centred therapy
    C. Family therapy
    D. Psychoanalytic psychotherapy
    E. Rational emotive therapy

69. The ABCD system of emotional self-control is a feature of which of the following therapies?

    A. Client-centred therapy
    B. Cognitive therapy
    C. Family therapy
    D. Psychoanalytic psychotherapy
    E. Rational emotive behaviour therapy

70. **Behavioural activation can be used as a method of treating depression. In behavioural activation, one's day is structured with certain activities consistent with the intended positive outcome. Which of the following is the major component of activity scheduling?**

    A. Keeping notes and diaries to prompt the patient
    B. Listing only pleasurable activities on the schedule
    C. Negative reinforcement of avoidance behaviour
    D. Postponing an activity until the development of full motivation
    E. Scheduling activities that have been avoided

1. C.   Various methods are used to measure the attitudes of a subject on a specific issue. The method described in Question 1 is an example of the Thurstone scale. When constructing a Thurstone scale, hundreds of statements are initially produced pertaining to a particular topic, for example abortion. These statements are presented to a sample of people (similar to a panel of judges) who are asked to score the statements on an 11-point scale. A set number of statements, for example 10 on each extreme (positive and negative attitude), are chosen based on the consistency of scores given by the judges. Each of these statements will carry a value that is the average of 100 judgements on the 11-point scale. These 20 statements are clubbed together to produce an attitude scale, which is administered to the subject. The subject will then indicate what statements he agrees with. It is not often used because the method is too tedious. The 11 points (used to rate each statement) are assumed to be intervals and averages are used to obtain the value scores. This is not entirely accurate as the 11-point scale is in fact ordinal. In the Likert scale, graded 'strongly agree' to 'strongly disagree' measures are employed. It is statistically reliable (ordinal data) and easy to construct. It is usually constructed as a five- to seven-point scale.

Thambirajah MS. *Psychological Basis of Psychiatry*. Elsevier, 2005, p. 192.

2. A.   Contrary to popular belief, the group that is paid more will not appreciate the boring task. As they obtained a good incentive, they will not develop a dissonance. They may lie about its usefulness but in fact they will not change their belief about the boring nature of the task. In contrast, the lowly paid group will experience a cognitive dissonance between the two facts— 'This task is boring' and 'I am doing this task without much incentive'. Hence they will change their initial attitude towards the task and, in fact, will start liking the task. This is called the one-dollar/ 20-dollar experiment and explains processes that substantiate counter-attitudinal behaviours.

Gross R. *Psychology: The Science of Mind and Behaviour*, 5th edn. Hodder Arnold, 2005, p. 420.

3. D.   In the field of attitude research, the relative lack of correlation between expressed attitude and actual behaviour is an important hurdle. Attitudes can be elicited with specific assessment of:
1. The target of one's attitude
2. The actual action expected when faced with the target
3. The specified context in which such action is expected
4. The time when this action is expected.
With such specific assessment, the correlation between measured attitude and behaviour improves considerably. Single instances of behaviours are not reliable indicators of attitudes. Repeated observations of behaviours (not measurement of attitudes, as stated in Choice A) may improve the validity. The notion that a specific behaviour is influenced by one predominant attitude is too simple and reductionist. Various attitudes interact to produce behaviour. There is no evidence to suggest that a postal survey of attitudes has better validity than other methods.

Gross R. *Psychology: The Science of Mind and Behaviour*, 5th edn. Hodder Arnold, 2005, p. 410.

4.A.   The success of persuasive communication depends on many variables. These variables can be grouped as those that depend on the source (communicator—the politician in this case), the message itself, the audience, and the medium of communication. A communicator who is perceived to be reliable, likeable, attractive, and an expert are positive features that will result in effective persuasion. When the audience perceive a degree of similarity with the communicator, the effectiveness of persuasion increases. Inducing moderate but not a high degree of fear can help effective persuasion. When a message is presented to a well-educated and highly informed audience who will hear both sides of a story before making a judgement, explaining both pros and cons (two-sided messages) is more useful than just highlighting the advantages of a policy (one-sided messages). Providing disclaimers, for example highlighting one's distance from the advocated message, is often counterproductive.

Thambirajah MS. *Psychological Basis of Psychiatry*. Elsevier, 2005, pp. 225–226.

5.D.   The relationship between fear and persuasion is an inverted U shape—too little or too much fear will reduce the effectiveness of persuasion. This is similar to the Yerkes–Dodson law which correlates arousal with performance of an activity. When one is too aroused, performance is inhibited. At the same time, when someone is not aroused at all, performance is again inhibited. Optimum arousal seems to be necessary for peak performances. This is clearly evident in performing sexual activity. When a subject is made to feel vulnerable, this increases one's concerns and, as a result, increases one's attention to a message. For example in order to persuade adolescents to practice safer sex, the high prevalence of HIV is highlighted before advising safe sexual practices.

Thambirajah MS. *Psychological Basis of Psychiatry*. Elsevier, 2005, p. 225.

6.A.   Shaping refers to an operant conditioning technique that has been used in autistic children. It consists of successive reinforcement of behaviours that approximate to the final desired behaviour. It is different from chaining in that chaining involves eliciting a complex behaviour by reinforcing the comparatively simpler components of the behavioural chain. Flooding is a behavioural technique used in exposure therapy. In this technique, sudden exposure to highly threatening stimulus (from a hierarchical list of various anxiety provoking situations) is attempted. It is often unacceptable to many patients and is not popular. Aversion therapy is not used in present-day behavioural treatment. It refers to a conditioning technique where negative reinforcement is used to bring about a desired behaviour or to stop an unwanted behaviour. It is not very effective as any positive outcome tends to be temporary. Token economy is a contingency technique where immediately available secondary reinforcers (e.g. coupons, vouchers, tokens) are used to reward a desirable behaviour. Later, primary reinforcers can be obtained in exchange for secondary reinforcers. A wide variety of behaviours can be thus reinforced even in large group settings.

Gross R. *Psychology: The Science of Mind and Behaviour*, 5th edn. Hodder Arnold, 2005, p. 822.

7. A. This is an example of cognitive dissonance or, more precisely, attitude behaviour discrepancy. Cognitive dissonance is defined as a psychological tension that arises when inconsistent cognitions are held simultaneously. A similar tension can also occur when there is a discrepancy between one's attitude and behaviour. When one is faced with such dissonance, a change in behaviour happens very rarely. Changing one's behaviour requires more motivation, effort, and sustained energy. Instead one of the following three happens more often:

1. Removal or denial of the dissonant cognition ('There is no evidence that smoking is harmful')
2. Trivializing the dissonant cognition ('I do not smoke that much' or 'Pleasure is more important than health')
3. Adding a new consonant cognition to counter balance the dissonance ('Smoking helps to reduce my tension' or 'Not everyone who smokes will die early').

Thambirajah MS. *Psychological Basis of Psychiatry*. Elsevier, 2005, p. 222.

8. D. The concept of cognitive dissonance is therapeutically employed in motivation enhancement therapy. When treating harmful users of alcohol, the evidence for harm caused by alcohol is highlighted along with reflecting on one's continuous drinking behaviour. This induces a cognitive dissonance which will drive towards an action.

Thambirajah MS. *Psychological Basis of Psychiatry*. Elsevier, 2005, p. 224.

9. C. Self-esteem refers to an evaluative stand one holds about oneself. In self-psychology an array of terms are used, somewhat confusing the concepts.

Self-consciousness: awareness of distinct self compared to other objects in the environment. Only humans are thought to possess full self-consciousness.

Self-image: this refers to an answer one might give for the question 'who are you?' It includes one's description of social roles (social self), personality traits, and physical characters (bodily self). We do not feel odd swallowing our own saliva as it is a part of our self-image. Imagine being asked to swallow someone else's saliva!

Self-esteem: this refers to a personal judgement of worthiness expressed in the attitudes one holds towards oneself.

Ideal-self: this represents 'what we would like ourselves to be'. One's self-esteem depends on the discrepancy between one's ideal self and self-image.

Gross R. *Psychology: The Science of Mind and Behaviour*, 5th edn. Hodder Arnold, 2005, p. 568.

10. A. Behavioural couples therapy is a specific intervention for alcoholism. It is derived from a general behavioural conceptualization of substance abuse, which assumes that family interactions reinforce alcohol-seeking behaviour. It has strong empirical and randomized controlled trial-based evidence for its effectiveness. It encourages family members to reward abstinence. Soon after the substance user seeks help, the patient and their partner are seen together in therapy for 15 to 20 out-patient couple sessions over 5 to 6 months. The therapist arranges a daily 'sobriety contract' in which the patient states his or her intent not to drink or use drugs that day (traditionally, one day at a time), and the spouse expresses support for the patient's efforts to stay abstinent. Stop–start or squeeze–pause techniques (Masters and Johnson) are used for premature ejaculation. Sex offender treatment programmes in the UK largely use Cognitive Behavioural Therapy (CBT)-based treatment approaches.

Fals-Stewart W and Birchler GR. A national survey of the use of couples therapy in substance abuse treatment. *Journal of Substance Abuse Treatment* 2001; **20**: 277–283.

11. E.   All of the given factors in the question play equally important roles in developing one's self-concept. Parents react differently to their children according to their birth order. The eldest born is given more responsibility. This leads to a higher self-esteem in most first-born children. In a social environment, individuals make constant comparisons with other persons surrounding them in different domains. One's self-concept depends very much on the outcome of such comparisons. As one grows older, one takes up a variety of social roles. The role we play in society is crucial in the development of self-concept. Individuals often identify themselves as a part of a group for example 'I am a football fan'. This social identity plays an important role in self-development.

Gross R. *Psychology: The Science of Mind and Behaviour*, 5th edn. Hodder Arnold, 2005, p. 573.

12. A.   Various theories have been put forward to explain prejudice and discrimination. According to relative deprivation theory, when sudden discrepancies develop between the needs of a society and resources possessed by the society, acute relative deprivation results. This in turn leads to aggressive and discriminatory behaviour against a specific target, even though the targeted group was in no way responsible for the deprivation. Group membership theory states that mere perception of the existence of another group is sufficient to trigger discriminatory behaviour. Prejudice is common in individuals who suffer excessive disciplinary upbringing and later develop authoritarian personality. However, this authoritarian personality theory fails to explain sudden surges in social prejudice. According to social identity theory an individual strives to achieve a positive self-esteem by improving his social identity. Positive preference to one's own group (in group) can improve this image. Prejudice and discrimination can develop from this biased attitude. Cognitive dissonance theory is not a theory of prejudice.

Gross R. *Psychology: The Science of Mind and Behaviour*, 5th edn. Hodder Arnold, 2005, p. 427–429.

13. B.   Personality theories can be broadly divided into nomothetic theories and idiographic theories. Nomothetic theories take the view that there are common underlying traits in people's personality; we only differ in the degree (and intensity) to which we have these various traits. Cattell and Eysenck are important proponents of this approach. Idiographic theories take the view that every individual is unique and we cannot place people into boxes of similar shape and size. Psychoanalytic theories of personality and humanistic theories are examples of idiographic approach. According to idiographic theories, personality is better described than measured. Personality is thought to be pathoplastic, as it modifies psychiatric disease expression and itself becomes modified by the influence of a disease process. Ambiguous stimuli elicit responses that are coloured by one's personality and style of thinking. Projective tests, such as Rorschach's ink blot test, utilize this property.

Thambirajah MS. *Psychological Basis of Psychiatry*. Elsevier, 2005, p. 64.

14. C.   Prejudice is best viewed as an attitude whose components include a cognitive part (stereotypes), affective part (hostility and hatred), and behavioural part. The behaviour related to prejudice can vary from mild to a severe extreme. Allport described (i) antilocution, (ii) avoidance of contact, (iii) discrimination, (iv) physical attack, and (v) extermination, as the behaviours associated with prejudice. One can have positive, neutral, or negative prejudice too. Of note is the term racism, which refers to an economical and political ideology while racial prejudice refers to individual attitudes.

Gross R. *Psychology: The Science of Mind and Behaviour*, 5th edn. Hodder Arnold, 2005, p. 424.

15. C. Theory of mind develops around the age of 3 1/2 to 4 years old in most humans. Initially this is confined to the rudimentary concept of private thinking—understanding that one's thoughts are not visible to others. This is followed by understanding the existence of similar mental processes in other individuals—termed theory of mind. False belief task or Sally Anne task is used to test the theory of mind.

Gross R. *Psychology: The Science of Mind and Behaviour*, 5th edn. Hodder Arnold, 2005, p. 576.

16. E. Age is often the first social category learnt by a child. It is thought to be developed even before a child develops full language abilities. Even the concept of numbers comes later. Exemplifying this, it is noted that age-related mistakes, such as calling an adult a baby, almost never occur in children. Gender identity develops around 3 years of age.

Gross R. *Psychology: The Science of Mind and Behaviour*, 5th edn. Hodder Arnold, 2005, p. 576.

17. C. Self-recognition could be demonstrated in a growing infant by using a mirror. When a red dot is unknowingly placed on the face of a child, the child starts touching its face to explore the dot when a mirror is shown. This 'touching the dot' phenomenon does not occur less than 15 months of age; 5 to 25% of infants touch the dot by 18 months, while nearly 75% touch the dot by age 20 months. It is thus concluded that self-recognition rapidly develops between 18 and 20 months. Object permanence is thought to be a prerequisite to develop self-recognition so it is not possible before 9 months of age.

Gross R. *Psychology: The Science of Mind and Behaviour*, 5th edn. Hodder Arnold, 2005, p. 579.

18. C. Gallup conducted the famous 'touching the dot' experiments to demonstrate self-recognition. It is noted that only higher primates and humans older than 20 months successfully demonstrate 'touching the dot'. Mirror recognition by primates may be a reflection of behavioural recognition, that is 'the one in the mirror is the same as me' rather than self-recognition, that is 'the one in the mirror is me'.

Gross R. *Psychology: The Science of Mind and Behaviour*, 5th edn. Hodder Arnold, 2005, p. 576–577.

19. A. When we spend much effort in attaining a goal but do not attain the goal eventually, we are faced with a dissonance. The two facts 'I worked really hard' and 'I failed my exam' cannot coexist logically. Hence one starts perceiving that the result is not so bad and some may even consider that the result was indeed good for one's spiritual progress! This 'suffering-leads-to-liking' effect is also called effort justification dissonance. There is no narcissism or passive aggression in such behaviour. This is not a denial as the subject still accepts the failure but interprets it differently.

Thambirajah MS. *Psychological Basis of Psychiatry*. Elsevier, 2005, p. 224.

20. B. Osgood's Semantic Differential Scale is used to measure verbally expressed attitudes. It allows different attitudes about a particular topic to be measured on the same scale. It includes various factors constituting an attitude; for example while expressing one's attitudes regarding a politician one can rate him using an evaluative component (good ↔ bad), activity component (active ↔ inactive), and potency component (powerful ↔ weak), etc. Between the extremes of these bipolar adjectives a seven-point scale is placed and the subject is asked to indicate a score for each factor. Osgood's semantic differential assumes that every concept can be represented in a hypothetical semantic space with two extremes. Sociometry is a method of measuring interpersonal attitudes and it involves constructing a sociogram—for example a representation of 'who likes whom' in a family. Guttman's scalogram consists of various statements arranged in a hierarchy. Choosing a statement invariably implies that all statements that come below the chosen statement are accepted. Scalogram is also utilized in measurement of attitudes.

Thambirajah MS. *Psychological Basis of Psychiatry*. Elsevier, 2005, p. 192.

21. E.   Reciprocity negotiation, role reversal, and sculpting are terms associated with couples therapy. In reciprocity negotiation, mutual rewarding of desirable behaviours through expression of affection or approval is carried out. This is often a primary component in couples therapy. In role reversal, mutual exchange of viewpoints takes place in a role-play setting. This helps in understanding each other's differing points of view of an issue. This technique is also used in psychodrama and group therapy. Sculpting refers to silent enactment of positions that express an aspect of relationship without verbal exchanges. Socratic questioning and guided discovery are terms associated with cognitive therapy.

Gross R. *Psychology: The Science of Mind and Behaviour*, 5th edn. Hodder Arnold, 2005, p. 432, Key Study 25.1.

22. D.   In simple terms, repetition compulsion refers to a person's tendency to repeat past traumatic behaviours. In psychoanalysis, ego defences are considered to rein over id impulses. When this defence is superseded, conflict arises leading to anxiety and various defences invoked in response. The ego mediates between timely release of id impulses and morals imposed by the superego. At times, the direct control of superego is thwarted and id impulses repetitively present, that is repetition compulsion which is a form of acting out.

Sadock BJ and Sadock VA. *Kaplan and Sadock's Synopsis of Psychiatry: Behavioral Sciences/Clinical Psychiatry*, 10th edn. Lippincott Williams and Wilkins, 2007, p. 195.

23. D.   Regression refers to moving back on one's developmental behaviours at times of crisis, as exemplified in the question. Repression is the shifting of conscious conflicts to the unconscious, leading to reduced anxiety. Sadism is purposeful inflicting of pain on oneself.

Sadock BJ and Sadock VA. *Kaplan and Sadock's Synopsis of Psychiatry: Behavioral Sciences/Clinical Psychiatry*, 10th edn. Lippincott Williams and Wilkins, 2007, p. 197.

24. A.   Disintegration anxiety precedes other types of anxiety discussed in the question. According to Klein, soon after birth and thereafter the child experiences an intense fear of fragmentation, called disintegration anxiety by later theorists. This is sequentially followed by persecutory fear (against the mother) and, later, separation anxiety. Castration anxiety is seen in the oedipal stage. Superego anxiety is the anxiety arising out of choices one has to make between instinctual drives and social morals. This is a mature type of anxiety that develops late in a child.

Gelder MG *et al.*, eds. *New Oxford Textbook of Psychiatry*. Oxford University Press, 2000, p. 370.

25. A.   Jung was widely expected to succeed Freud as the leader of psychoanalysis, but Jung distanced himself from Freud on the account of Freud's ideas on infantile sexuality. Jung founded analytical psychology and expanded on 'unconscious' to include 'collective unconscious'. Jungian psychotherapy is a classical psychoanalytic therapy in the broad sense but Jung introduced active imagination or fantasy as a mode of therapy. He emphasized having holidays from analysis to reflect and think. He encouraged art therapy too. He stressed the concept of individuation. Thanatos is not a predominant Jungian concept and it is not an objects relation therapy.

Gelder MG *et al.*, eds. *New Oxford Textbook of Psychiatry*. Oxford University Press, 2000, p. 346.

26. D.   This example refers to rationalization. A rationalizing individual offers rational explanations in an attempt to justify unacceptable attitudes or beliefs or actions. Intellectualization is closely allied to rationalization, but it is very important to note that in rationalization, the motives are usually primal and instinctually determined, for example sex, aggression, greed, etc. Intellectualization is an immature defence. It refers to excessively using intellectual processes to avoid experiencing painful emotions (not necessarily libidinal). An intellectualizing individual places undue emphasis on inanimate objects or parts to avoid dealing with emotion-provoking, 'living' elements. He may have more focus on outside reality to avoid inner feelings; in the process he may pay more attention to irrelevant details.

Sadock BJ and Sadock VA. *Kaplan and Sadock's Synopsis of Psychiatry: Behavioral Sciences/Clinical Psychiatry*, 10th edn. Lippincott Williams and Wilkins, 2007, p. 205.

27. D.   Cathexis refers to the supposed libidinal energy stored in neurones and kept under control by the monitoring action of ego. Release of cathexis presents as impulses and defence mechanisms serve to alter the expression. Libidinal energy may be constructive sexual energy or destructive aggression. The junction between two neurones is called a synapse. Re-enactment of childhood conflicts during a therapy session refers to transference. Dream work includes various processes and revisions and not defence mechanisms as such.

Sadock BJ and Sadock VA. *Kaplan and Sadock's Synopsis of Psychiatry: Behavioral Sciences/Clinical Psychiatry*, 10th edn. Lippincott Williams and Wilkins, 2007, p. 193.

28. B.   Transference neurosis involves the re-creation of the patient's conflicts enacted within the psychoanalysis session. This enactment mirrors aspects of the infantile neurosis. The transference neurosis usually develops in the middle phase of analysis, when the patient, after initial engagement, stops displaying consistent motivation but engages in therapy to attain emotional satisfaction of re-enacting her infantile conflict. Emergence of the transference neurosis is usually a slow and gradual process but when a patient has a propensity for transference regression (e.g. emotionally unstable or histrionic) this can occur quiet early in the therapy.

Sadock BJ and Sadock VA. *Kaplan and Sadock's Synopsis of Psychiatry: Behavioral Sciences/Clinical Psychiatry*, 10th edn. Lippincott Williams and Wilkins, 2007, p. 206.

29. C.   Self–object relationship is the central theme in object relations theory propounded by Melanie Klein. The relationship between the internal and external world as represented by objects is studied in detail by object relation therapists. The relationship between past and present is emphasized more in a Freudian style of psychoanalysis.

Gelder MG *et al.*, eds. *New Oxford Textbook of Psychiatry*. Oxford University Press, 2000, p. 349.

30. C.   Preference towards one's own group with positive in-group attributional bias helps in preserving one's social identity. According to social identity theory (SIT), an individual strives to achieve a positive self-esteem through personal and also social identity. So both exist concurrently. One can have several social identities according to the community in which one lives. Social identity has direct influence on one's self-esteem. By improving one's social identity, one can improve self-esteem. Unfortunately, while developing a strong social identity, in addition to pro in-group bias, one develops anti out-group bias that results in discrimination.

Gross R. *Psychology: The Science of Mind and Behaviour*, 5th edn. Hodder Arnold, 2005, p. 433.

31. C.   Corrective emotional experience was seen by Alexander as the central part of change secondary to psychotherapy. Processes that take place in a therapy setting give the patient an opportunity to reflect on their past experiences and make necessary behavioural or cognitive and emotional changes to reduce one's difficulties. Positive identification refers to an unconscious group mechanism in which a person incorporates the characteristics and the qualities of the group. Catharsis refers to the process by which mere expression of ideas and conflicts is accompanied by an emotional response which produces a sense of relief. Group cohesion refers to the sense that the group is working together towards a common goal.

Sadock BJ and Sadock VA. *Kaplan and Sadock's Synopsis of Psychiatry: Behavioral Sciences/Clinical Psychiatry*, 10th edn. Lippincott Williams and Wilkins, 2007, p. 937.

32. D.   Yalom cited 11 'curative' factors responsible for change in groups. Stability of administration is not one of them. The curative factors include instillation of hope, universality, imparting information (feedback), altruism, corrective recapitulation, socialization techniques, imitative behaviour, interpersonal learning, group cohesiveness, catharsis, and existential factors. Of these, cohesiveness and learning from feedback are valued positively, though other factors may also be important.

Gelder MG *et al.*, eds. *New Oxford Textbook of Psychiatry*. Oxford University Press, 2000, pp. 1452 and 1448.

33. D.   The term protagonist in therapeutic dramatization (psychodrama) refers to the patient. Auxiliary ego refers to an accomplice who acts as a significant person in patient's life. The director is the therapist who conducts the role playing.

Sadock BJ and Sadock VA. *Kaplan and Sadock's Synopsis of Psychiatry: Behavioral Sciences/Clinical Psychiatry*, 10th edn. Lippincott Williams and Wilkins, 2007, p. 939.

34. B.   According to Freud, id is the most primitive structure to develop. A baby is more or less born with the pleasure principle id. Soon after birth the child develops a concept of internal self versus external world, coinciding with the development of ego. Superego is largely a by-product of introjected parental values and social discipline. This develops only when a child is able to identify with its same-sex parent. This takes place following successful resolution of the oedipal complex. Interestingly, Freud considered the superego of girls to be weaker than boys as oedipal complex develops in a different trajectory for girls. A girl believes she has been castrated by her mother during development. She develops 'penis envy' and loves her father but, realizing she cannot have a penis, she replaces the envy with a wish for a baby. This leads to identification with her mother—but as prominent conflict-related anxiety is not involved, superego that develops at resolution of the Electra complex is weaker compared to boys.

Thambirajah MS. *Psychological Basis of Psychiatry*. Elsevier, 2005, p. 329.

35. D.   According to psychodynamic theory, different phases of development are associated with different levels of anxiety. As soon as a child is born, he/she experiences what Klein described as disintegration anxiety, followed by persecutory (destructive) anxiety against the mother with resultant separation anxiety (related to depressive position). Here the fear is one of losing the loved object, that is the mother. In the oedipal phase, the most daunting fear is castration anxiety. When maturing out of the oedipal stage and entering the latent or genital stage, the child learns the experience of guilt secondary to development of superego. Hence development of superego needs resolution of oedipal conflict.

Gelder MG *et al.*, eds. *New Oxford Textbook of Psychiatry*. Oxford University Press, 2000, p. 370, Table 3.

36. C. The technique of paradoxical injunction developed from work of Gregory Bateson. Here, a therapist suggests that the patient intentionally engages in the unwanted behaviour, as described in the question. Though this seems to be counterintuitive, the therapy can create new insights for some patients. It is sometimes used in family therapy. Triangulation is one of the processes concerning family dynamics wherein the child is roped into conflicts between the mother and father and a triad is sustained. Reframing is also called positive connotation. It refers to redefining and relabelling all negatively expressed feelings and behaviours as positive. It is used in family therapy. Covert sensitization refers to a behavioural method of reducing the frequency of unwanted behaviour by associating it with the imagination (covert) of unpleasant consequences.

Sadock BJ and Sadock VA. *Kaplan and Sadock's Synopsis of Psychiatry: Behavioral Sciences/Clinical Psychiatry*, 10th edn. Lippincott Williams and Wilkins, 2007, pp. 142 and 943.

37. D. Group therapies can be classified according to the objectives of the group and how the group is led or managed (leadership). Highly specific, target-oriented groups include structured groups for drug use or alcohol use, activity groups such as occupational therapy groups, etc. These groups have a high level of leader input. Psychodrama, music therapy, and systems-centred groups are some less-specific therapies but are highly directed by the leader or therapist. Problem-solving therapy and psychoeducational groups are highly specific but have a low level of therapist activity. Support groups, art therapy, interpersonal therapy, and groups such as Tavistock-model analytic groups have a low level of leader activity and have low specificity with respect to treatment goals.

Gelder MG *et al.*, eds. *New Oxford Textbook of Psychiatry*. Oxford University Press, 2000, p. 1442.

38. D. Various defence mechanisms are used by patients and so-called normal populations at different times. People can have a style or pattern of predominant defence mechanisms. Traditionally, the psychodynamic school has proposed certain defences to be associated with certain diseases: obsessive compulsive disorder (OCD) with isolation of affect, undoing, and reaction formation; anorexia with denial, displacement, and rationalization; hysteria with conversion and repression; somatoform disorders with somatization; fugue with dissociation; schizoid personality with fantasy; borderline personality with splitting, projective identification, and introjection.

Thambirajah MS. *Psychological Basis of Psychiatry*. Elsevier, 2005, pp. 335–336.

39. D. The four major principles on which a therapeutic community is based are exemplified by the Henderson hospital model. According to this model, the major components (with a mnemonic CPD-R) are:
1. Communalism—staff are not separated from inmates by uniforms or behaviours; mutual helping and learning occurs
2. Permissiveness—tolerating each other and realizing unpredictable behaviour can happen within the community
3. Democratization—shared decision making and joint running of the unit
4. Reality confrontation—self-deception or distortions from reality are dealt with honestly and openly by all members without formalities.

Instillation of hope is necessary for any supportive psychotherapy but has not been described as one of the four major principles behind therapeutic communities.

Gelder MG *et al.*, eds. *Shorter Oxford Textbook of Psychiatry*, 5th edn. Oxford University Press, 2006, p. 608, Box 22.8.

40. B. Social psychologists have put forward various explanations to answer the question 'how to reduce prejudice?' Allport developed the 'contact hypothesis' to explain that when people of equal social status stay in close contact and pursue a common goal, the differences between them can disappear. It is well established that 'autistic hostility' between members of two groups exists due to lack of sufficient knowledge about the members of the opposite group. This ignorance leads to reinforcement of negative stereotypes, for example 'We are hard working; they are lazy'. This is also known as a 'mirror-image phenomenon'. The assumption that everyone in the opposite group is the same, called 'illusion of out-group homogeneity', also reduces with improved social contact, but it is important to note that this does not relate to a necessary increase in personal friendships between opposite group members. Imposing strongly one-sided conditions for negotiations will reduce perceived equality status, leading to maintenance of prejudice. Self-experience of prejudice by the members of one group can reduce the prejudiced behaviour exhibited by these members towards others. This was demonstrated by Elliott in the blue eyes/brown eyes experiment. When groups are set common goals to pursue, cooperation instead of competition ensues. This aids in reducing prejudice.

Gross R. *Psychology: The Science of Mind and Behaviour*, 5th edn. Hodder Arnold, 2005, p. 438.

41. B. The description in Question 41 refers to 'holding'. Holding was proposed by Winnicot. While administering psychotherapy, the affective and cognitive dispositions of a therapist play an important part. The cognitive capacity of the therapist to maintain objectivity and focus on selected facts during a discourse is called 'containing' (proposed by Bion). The affective disposition of the therapist, which helps in restraining oneself from retaliating to negative transferences, is called 'holding'. Working through refers to the process by which the therapist repeatedly elaborates the identified conflict throughout the therapy in order to enable the patient to recognize and deal with it effectively.

Gelder MG *et al.*, eds. *New Oxford Textbook of Psychiatry*. Oxford University Press, 2000, p. 351.

42. D. Patients must be abstinent at the time of initiation of acamprosate. In precontemplation phase the patient will simply refuse an intervention. While contemplating treatment the patient will be still drinking actively. When he acts to stop drinking he will need withdrawal support. This is the best time to start acamprosate so that he can have reduced craving, which will aid him to stay in maintenance mode and reduce the likelihood of relapses. An occasional single relapse need not result in discontinuation of acamprosate. Starting when the patient had already relapsed will not be an ideal strategy.

Mason BJ. Treatment of alcohol-dependent outpatients with acamprosate: a clinical review. *Journal of Clinical Psychiatry* 2001; **62** (Suppl. 20): 42–48.

43. B. This question tests one's knowledge about Main's Adult Attachment Interview. This is a 15-item, semistructured, psychodynamic interview of adults exploring one's experience as a child. The attachment style one had as a child correlates with the type of responses given when answering this interview. Those who had secure attachment provide spontaneous and coherent answers with an ability to talk freely about negative experiences in childhood. Those who had an avoidant (insecure) pattern often minimize their experiences, do not elaborate on them, and do not use colourful metaphors during the discourse. Those who had insecure but ambivalent (enmeshed) attachment use multiple emotionally laden responses and ramble excessively. Broken continuity and interrupted logical flow of thoughts is seen in those who had insecure, disorganized attachment pattern. Multiple attachments are common and their presence can be detected without the need for a discourse analysis.

Gelder MG *et al.*, eds. *New Oxford Textbook of Psychiatry*. Oxford University Press, 2000, p. 352.

44. C. Interpersonal psychotherapy (IPT) was proposed by Klerman and Weissman. The theory behind IPT is the observation that the development and maintenance of depression occur in a social and interpersonal context. The outcomes of most psychiatric illnesses are influenced by the interpersonal relationships between the patient and significant others. The therapy takes place in three phases: identification of problems, targeted action, and consolidating gains. Major interpersonal problems can be classified as grief, role deficits, role disputes, and role transitions. Grief refers to loss of a relationship. Role dispute arises due to conflicts between the related individuals. Role transition refers to life changes, for example change in job, etc. Deficit refers to social impoverishment and inadequate relationships.

Sadock BJ and Sadock VA. *Kaplan and Sadock's Synopsis of Psychiatry: Behavioral Sciences/Clinical Psychiatry*, 10th edn. Lippincott Williams and Wilkins, 2007, p. 966.

45. D. These terms are used in cognitive analytical therapy (CAT), founded by Ryle. CAT views behaviour in terms of a procedural sequence model. When a goal-directed activity is carried out, a sequence of mental components is involved. An important function is making and testing hypotheses for successful social interactions. Some times, in what are termed neurotic repetitions, these sequences fail and effective hypothesis testing does not take place. These are:
1. Traps: where negative assumptions lead to blunting of the hypothetical approach
2. Dilemmas: false dichotomies are identified in decision making wherein the tested hypothesis can have either of just two outcomes
3. Snags (or subtle negative aspect of goals): in spite of having a good hypothesis this does not get tested as it is perceived to be forbidden or dangerous.

Denman C. Cognitive–analytic therapy. *Advances in Psychiatric Treatment* 2001; **7**: 243–256.

46. A. Dialectical behaviour therapy (DBT) was specifically designed by Linehan to address repeated self-harm behaviour, especially in patients with emotional instability. The core components of DBT are:
1. Affect regulation
2. Distress tolerance
3. Social skills training
4. Enhancing interpersonal effectiveness.
Ellis developed rational emotive therapy, which is predominantly cognitive-theory based.

Linehan M. *Skills Training Manual for Treating Borderline Personality Disorder*. Guilford Press, 1993.

47. B. This is called reciprocal inhibition. Wolpe introduced this term to explain how contradictory and incompatible responses cannot be conditioned to coexist simultaneously; as a result one response will be suppressed. In this example, suppression of stranger anxiety response (barking) follows the evocation of faithfulness and friendliness in the presence of the dog's primary food-giver. The physiologically antagonistic response of friendliness serves to extinguish barking through reciprocal inhibition. Reciprocal determinism and vicarious learning refer to social learning or modelling theory. There was no applied relaxation or biofeedback provided to the dog in question.

Thambirajah MS. *Psychological Basis of Psychiatry*. Elsevier, 2005, p. 9.

48. D. This question tests one's knowledge of Beck's cognitive distortions. Cognitive distortions are dysfunctional patterns of thinking that serve to produce and maintain depression or anxiety. A useful mnemonic to remember cognitive distortions is MOSPAD—minimization or magnification, overgeneralization, selective abstraction, personalization, arbitrary inference, and dichotomous thinking. In this scenario, the teacher can see one sleepy student amidst many active participants, yet the teacher chooses to select the negative aspect of the truth—selective abstraction. In arbitrary inference one comes to conclusion without seeing both sides of a coin. In minimization, one downplays one's successful achievements. Magnification reefers to overrating one's negative aspects. In dichotomous thinking, a subject splits events around him to 'black or white', that is either good or bad with no grey area in between. Catastrophic interpretation is seen in panic attacks where minor events are misinterpreted in catastrophic proportions.

Thambirajah MS. *Psychological Basis of Psychiatry*. Elsevier, 2005, p. 149.

49. D. Babbling refers to the repetitive production of consonants around the age of 6 months. It is seen at the same developmental age irrespective of one's culture and mother tongue. It is largely an innate developmental milestone. Even deaf and mute children babble, but around 9 to 12 months this reduces and stops. Normally, babbling continues well into 18 months of age and does not stop with the production of the first words. Babbling is practiced alone by a child even in the absence of any adults; this means that communication is not the only intention in babbling.

Gross R. *Psychology: The Science of Mind and Behaviour*, 5th edn. Hodder Arnold, 2005, p. 322, Box 19.1.

50. C. Source traits refer to those traits that act as basic building blocks of personality, as measured by Cattell's 16PF. Surface traits are easily observable traits that are correlated strongly with one another but are not important for making one's personality. Allport derived various trait labels from around 18 000 adjectives used in English. According to him, there are three main variants of traits—cardinal traits are the influential, core traits while central traits refer to the five to 10 less general traits an individual possesses. Least important of all are secondary traits, which are least general and consistent and are only noticed by close friends.

Gross R. *Psychology: The Science of Mind and Behaviour*, 5th edn. Hodder Arnold, 2005, p. 741.

51. E. Kohlberg's stages of moral development include three major levels (which are not necessarily progressive phases during development), each containing two parts. In the stage of preconventional morality the child is initially punishment avoidant, that is anything that avoids punishment is a right thing to do. Later, reward orientation develops—anything that results in 'candies', as in this question, is morally right. In conventional morality, the child believes that the majority is always right and what pleases others must be morally right. Later, the child learns that doing one's duty and maintaining order defines moral values. The third level is one of postconventional mortality. Here, one thinks that an individual's life comes above all man-made laws and, if necessary, laws should be changed by mutual agreement in a democratic country. Some people develop a higher, stage 6 morality, called universal ethical orientation. Here, universal moral principles are upheld more than an individual's sense of personal right or wrong.

Gross R. *Psychology: The Science of Mind and Behaviour*, 5th edn. Hodder Arnold, 2005, p. 610, Box 35.5.

52. A. Freud observed that some patients became unwell when they started recovering from their difficulties during psychotherapy. He attributed this phenomenon to the guilt surrounding the change. This is usually noted in the middle phase of treatment. This must be differentiated from negative transference where aggressive or paranoid projective transference takes place, sometimes hindering the therapy progression. Termination reaction refers to the resistance offered by some patients while terminating therapy. The above example cannot be resistance to change as initial improvement could not have occurred as described if there was resistance to change.

Gelder MG *et al.*, eds. *New Oxford Textbook of Psychiatry*. Oxford University Press, 2000, p.1439.

53. E. Albert Bandura proposed the social learning theory based on modelling (vicarious learning). Cognitive variables are crucial in mediating social learning. These variables are:
1. Attention
2. Visual image or semantic code recorded in memory
3. Memory permanence using rehearsal and organization (retention)
4. Copying or imitation of behaviour
5. Motivation to perform the learnt act.
It is important to note that social learning differentiated learning from performance. Reinforcement is generally not needed for learning but for performance. Problem solving is not a cognitive variable mediating vicarious learning.

Gross R. *Psychology: The Science of Mind and Behaviour*, 5th edn. Hodder Arnold, 2005, p. 617, Box 35.7.

54. B. Supportive psychotherapy refers to a common component in many therapeutic operations. It refers to a supportive, explicitly reassuring approach to allay anxiety and help patients in crises. Positive instillation of hope, strengthening existing ego defence mechanisms, and environmental manipulation for supporting one's coping strategies are important components of supportive psychotherapy. It is generally provided unlimited in a predictable 'as and when necessary' manner. It is not specifically goal-oriented and hence social skills training cannot be considered as supportive psychotherapy.

Sadock BJ and Sadock VA. *Kaplan and Sadock's Synopsis of Psychiatry: Behavioral Sciences/Clinical Psychiatry*, 10th edn. Lippincott Williams and Wilkins, 2007, p. 929.

55. A. Catastrophic thinking is a common cognitive distortion seen in patients with panic attacks. Minor physiological aberrations, such as missed heart beats or palpitations are common events. A catastrophic thinker interprets these minor aberrations in catastrophic proportion, making him think he is going to have a heart attack or he is going to die. When a similar experience occurs with faintness or dizziness, this is interpreted as 'going crazy'. Secondary to such catastrophic thinking, autonomic arousal and resultant panic sets in.

Thambirajah MS. *Psychological Basis of Psychiatry*. Elsevier, 2005, p. 149.

56. B. Milgram conducted controversial experiments to explore why many conscientious individuals in Nazi Germany obeyed Hitler. In his paradigm, subjects were asked to administer a (sham) electric shock to a victim under some false pretence by pressing a dial. The victim can cry in agony to the awe and shock of many subjects. It was noted that most subjects would obey an authoritative experimenter and administer shocks, especially if they are not in close proximity to the victim or if the authority is keeping a close watch on the subjects. Peer rebellion against the orders of experimenter reduced obedience while proxy administration increased obedience. When the subjects were given more responsibility regarding the pain inflicted on the victim, the obedience (administering shocks) decreased.

Gross R. *Psychology: The Science of Mind and Behaviour*, 5th edn. Hodder Arnold, 2005, p. 458, Box 27.1.

57. D. Group polarization refers to the phenomenon described in Question 57. There are various processes that influence individuals when making decisions as a part of a group. The group can make more risky decisions than those that an individual him/herself can. This is called risky shift. A group discussion process can strengthen average individual inclinations and polarize the group in the direction where most individuals were heading already. This is called group polarization. While making extreme decisions, the desire to agree with other members of a group can override rational judgment applicable in individual decision making. This is called groupthink. Conformity is a process whereby no explicit requirement is made to do a certain task, but peer influence and need for acceptance pushes one to carry out the task. Obedience refers to conditions where the individual is explicitly asked to do a task and this instruction comes from an authority.

Gross R. Psychology: *The Science of Mind and Behaviour*, 5th edn. Hodder Arnold, 2005, p. 453.

58. C. At 18 months of age, the number of words understood by the child will usually exceed the number of words that the child can produce. Initially, a child uses words in a contextual fashion, for example the word duck is used only when a toy duck is pushed face down on the floor. Later the words get decontextualized and used more generously. At one point during development, the child uses 'holophrases' which are single words substituting the function of a full sentence. Verbal use of language is learnt earlier than propositions such as 'to', 'as', etc. Telegraphic speech consists of using two or more connected words without functional elements such as conjunctions or propositions for example 'Papa go bye'. This occurs around 18 months of age.

Gross R. Psychology: *The Science of Mind and Behaviour*, 5th edn. Hodder Arnold, 2005, p. 324.

59. B. The technique described here is called stimulus control. This is often utilized in relapse prevention for drug users and also in compulsive behaviours such as hair pulling or skin picking. It is not usually employed as a stand-alone therapy but is provided in combination with other behavioural and cognitive techniques to control compulsive symptoms. Self-monitoring refers to keeping a logbook or diary of problem behaviour in order to reflect and work through the problem. Chaining is a behavioural technique where successive reinforcement of simple behaviours leads to learning of a complex behaviour. Negative practice is a behavioural technique used in tics and Tourette's syndrome. Exposure and response prevention is used to reduce compulsions in OCD where exposure to an anxiety-provoking situation is deliberately coupled with not responding in a problematic fashion, that is compulsive behaviours.

Van Minnen A. *et al.* Treatment of trichotillomania with behavioral therapy or fluoxetine: A randomized, waiting-list controlled study. *Archives of General Psychiatry* 2003; **60**: 517–522.

60. D. The treatment described here is EMDR—eye movement desensitization and reprocessing. This technique was serendipitously discovered by Shapiro. When repeated eye movements in a relaxed state are induced by the therapist, conscious recollection of traumatic material can be successfully combined with positive thoughts. This has been advocated and practised for post-traumatic stress disorder (PTSD). The three components are:
1. Imagined exposure
2. Cognitive reappraisal replacing negative thoughts with positive ones
3. Saccadic eye movements induced by the therapist.
The role of the latter is not clearly established and it does not compare well against simple exposure therapy.

Gelder MG et al., eds. *Shorter Oxford Textbook of Psychiatry*, 5th edn. Oxford University Press, 2006, p. 593.

61. B.   The Parental Bonding Instrument (PBI) is a self-report measure to be completed by those who are at least 16 years of age. The subjects are asked to score their parents on 25 attitudinal and behavioural items (each with a four-point Likert scale), as remembered during the first 16 years of the respondent's development. Hence it is prone to a high degree of recall bias. Potential sources of error include 'amnesia' of early childhood memories, pressure to appear 'conventional', or 'social', bias due to personality factors, trait characteristics, mood, and other psychopathology. The construct validity is also questionable.

Wilhelm K, Niven H, Parker G *et al.* The stability of the Parental Bonding Instrument over a 20-year period. *Psychological Medicine* 2005; **35**: 387–393.

62. E.   The five-areas approach for assessment in CBT was proposed by Williams; it is a jargon-free and easily accessible model of CBT for use in busy clinical settings. It allows the patient and therapist to understand the patient's symptoms in a deeper manner by exploring:
1. Situation, relationships, resources, and practical problems
2. Symptoms such as physical feelings
3. Behaviours and activity level
4. Thinking
5. Feelings, mood, and emotions.

Wright B, Williams C, and Garland A. Using the Five Areas cognitive-behavioural therapy model with psychiatric patients. *Advances in Psychiatric Treatment* 2002; **8**: 307–315.

63. A.   Active discouragement of work may be counter-therapeutic in most conditions. CBT does not adopt such prescriptive approach to problem solving. Exploring the patient's beliefs about his/her illness is an important part of assessment during CBT. Similarly, clear goal-setting can be therapeutic and has a role in motivating the patient. Homework tasks may include putting into practice what the patient learns during treatment sessions. Using the patient's own language can be helpful in enhancing therapeutic alliance and avoid misinterpretations during the therapeutic process.

Wright B, Williams C, and Garland A. Using the Five Areas cognitive-behavioural therapy model with psychiatric patients. *Advances in Psychiatric Treatment* 2002; **8**: 307–315.

64. B.   Classic psychoanalytic theory of depression compares depression with mourning. High dependence and ambivalence in relationships may predispose to depression after object loss. The object referred to in psychotherapy need not necessarily be one's parent; it can be any other person or even an inanimate but personally important object. Identification is an unconscious mechanism wherein the self tries to become the same as the lost object in some respect. In depression, identification occurs on the basis of sympathy, guilt, or longing to keep a relationship with the lost object. In addition, it is thought that an excessively harsh or envious superego can influence severity, chronicity, and refractoriness of depression. Such superego turns aggression and anxiety against the self.

Taylor D. Psychoanalytic and psychodynamic therapies for depression: the evidence base. *Advances in Psychiatric Treatment* 2008; **14**: 401–413.

65. B.   The 'basic assumptions' put forward by Bion are processes that need to be tackled effectively for group work to proceed. Bion postulated that when people meet in a group 'basic assumptions' become prominent. The basic assumptions include dependency (being passive and expecting the group leader to provide answers), pairing (coupling of idealized group members could lead to the birth of some creative answer to their problems), and fight–flight (the group's response to perceived threats to its existence from outside) reactions. Various techniques employed in group therapy include 'mirroring' (non-judgmental reflection of one's experience), 'amplification' (increase in emotional resonance by sharing), and 'catharsis' (supported ventilation of emotions). Within a group, processes such as scape-goating (e.g. blaming one member for lack of progress) or idealization of the therapist could occur. Similarly, unhealthy denigration could happen among team members. These are thought to be counter-therapeutic to the progress of the treatment.

Sadock BJ and Sadock VA. *Kaplan and Sadock's Synopsis of Psychiatry: Behavioral Sciences/Clinical Psychiatry*, 10th edn. Lippincott Williams and Wilkins, 2007, p. 215.

66. A.   Jung introduced the terms extraversion and introversion. He believed that people had different attitudes towards life in general. According to Jung, an extravert is primarily interested in the world of external objects, as depicted by Martin, who wants to be in the company of his friends. An introvert is mostly interested in what goes on within his own mind. Jung thought that both attitudes were necessary for a full comprehension of reality. Indeed, a number of people are what Jung referred to as ambiverts, but people are usually one-sided and tended to one or other extreme. The other concepts introduced by Jung include the concept of the collective unconscious, archetypes, animus, anima, and the shadow. Constitutional psychology is a theory, developed in the 1940s, by American psychologist William Herbert Sheldon. He associated body types with temperament. He divided people into three types: ectomorphs (ectoderm–skinny), mesomorphs (mesoderm–muscle), and endomorphs (gut–fatty). As such, Sheldon thought these body types correspond to certain temperaments that fit quite closely to popular stereotypes of the modern day. For the ease of recall—'the skinny nerd' (ectomorph), 'the jolly fat man' (endomorph), 'the slow-witted tough guy' (mesomorph). Most scientists consider this theory to be outdated.

Gelder M *et al. New Oxford Textbook of Psychiatry*. Oxford University Press, 2000, pp. 345–346.

67. C.   According to Erikson, older people may look back on their lives with a sense of panic and a feeling that time is running out and chances are used up. This can lead to anxiety disorders. A decline in physical function can contribute to various psychosomatic illness, hypochondriasis, and depression. People who are facing death may find it intolerable not to have been generative or had significant attachments in life. Integrity, according to Erikson, is characterized by an acceptance of life. Without this acceptance people feel a sense of despair, leading to severe depression and suicide in some cases. Generativity is the stage prior to the stage of integrity, between 40 and 65, failure of which leads to stagnation. Intimacy stage is seen between 20 and 40 years, where significant relationships are acquired. A failure of this stage leads to isolation. Identity versus role confusion is seen in the teen years, leading up to 20, during which the individual develops a sense of self.

Sadock BJ and Sadock VA. *Kaplan and Sadock's Synopsis of Psychiatry: Behavioral Sciences/Clinical Psychiatry*, 10th edn. Lippincott Williams and Wilkins, 2007, p. 210.

68. B.   Carl Rogers believed that people are born with a capacity to direct themselves towards a level of completeness called self-actualization. Rogers viewed personality as a dynamic phenomenon, which involves communications, relationships, and self-concepts and which changes regularly. He developed a treatment programme called client-centred psychotherapy. Here the therapist helps the client to achieve their self-actualization by producing an atmosphere conducive to it. The therapist holds the clients with unconditional positive regard, accepting him/her for what he/she is. He encouraged active listening, empathy, and non-directiveness, all principles which have been adopted by mainstream psychiatry. Other therapeutic practices include attention to the present, focus on clients' feelings, emphasis on process, trust in the potential and self-responsibility of clients, and a philosophy grounded in a positive attitude toward them, rather than a preconceived structure of treatment.

Sadock BJ and Sadock VA. *Kaplan and Sadock's Synopsis of Psychiatry: Behavioral Sciences/Clinical Psychiatry*, 10th edn. Lippincott Williams and Wilkins, 2007, p. 24.

69. E.   Rational emotive behaviour therapy was first developed by Albert Ellis, an American psychologist, in the 1950s. It can be considered one of the first forms of cognitive behaviour therapy. The therapy is based on the concept of how people's view of various events can affect the consequences. Typically, a situation (antecedent or A), triggers certain beliefs (B) about A. These beliefs, which are usually dysfunctional, lead to certain behavioural and emotional consequences (C), which are again dysfunctional.

A (antecedent) → B (Beliefs) → Consequences (C)

The therapy is directed towards identifying these faulty beliefs and disputing (D) these beliefs. These steps are not very dissimilar from cognitive behaviour therapy, developed by Aaron Beck a decade later.

Froggatt W. *A Brief Introduction To Rational Emotive Behaviour Therapy.* http://www.rational.org.nz/prof/docs/Intro-REBT.pdf. Accessed on 11/03/2009.

70. E.   Behavioural activation is a treatment for depression developed by Martell. It is now delivered largely as a part of other behavioural and cognitive psychotherapies for depression. Behavioural activation involves the development of activity scheduling; the main focus of activity scheduling is the use of avoided activities as a guide for daily scheduling and functional analysis of cognitive processes that involve avoidance.

Veale D. Behavioural activation for depression. *Advances in Psychiatric Treatment* 2008; **14**: 29–36.

1. On administration of an unknown dose of a new antipsychotic, a 55-year-old man develops extra pyramidal symptoms. The dose at which this effect appears would be established in which phase of clinical trials?

    A. Phase 1
    B. Phase 2
    C. Preclinical phase
    D. Phase 3
    E. Phase 4

2. Haloperidol is more potent than chlorpromazine. Potency of a therapeutic formulation refers to

    A. Strength of binding to receptors
    B. Duration of action at receptors
    C. Size of the dose required to produce an effect
    D. Elimination half-life of a drug
    E. Proportion of available receptors occupied by a drug

3. Absorption of orally administered drugs is affected by which of the following

    A. Intestinal transit
    B. Co-administered drugs
    C. P-glycoprotein
    D. Presence of food
    E. All of the above

4. Which of the following conditions predisposes to a higher rate of transport through the blood–brain barrier?

    A. Presence of ionized drug molecules
    B. Presence of protein-bound drug molecules
    C. Presence of water-soluble drug molecules
    D. Presence of inflamed meninges
    E. All of the above

5. A 72-year-old patient with bipolar illness experiences more side-effects when taking the same medication that he was prescribed 30 years ago, when he was 42 years old. Which of the following is a possible explanation?

    A. Reduced proportion of body fat
    B. Increased liver enzyme activity
    C. Increased renal clearance of drugs
    D. Increased protein-binding fraction
    E. All of the above

6. Which one of the following has partial agonistic activity as a major therapeutic mechanism?

    A. Propranalol
    B. Olanzapine
    C. Lithium
    D. Pindolol
    E. Carbamazepine

7. A 44-year-old in-patient, recently started on clozapine, develops exacerbation of chronic sinusitis and appears excessively drowsy. All of the following remedial measures might interfere with clozapine metabolism except

    A. Coffee
    B. Quitting smoking
    C. Amoxicillin
    D. Erythromycin
    E. Ciprofloxacin

8. Imipramine is a tricyclic antidepressant. Which one of the following is true with respect to imipramine?

    A. It acts synergistically with ECT.
    B. Imipramine has no effect in atypical depression.
    C. Imipramine and CBT are equally effective in severe depression.
    D. Imipramine decreases non-REM sleep.
    E. Imipramine is not toxic in overdose.

9. Use of stimulants is relatively contraindicated in which of the following patients with ADHD?

    A. 9-year-old child with a family history of ADHD
    B. 9-year-old child with a family history of psychosis
    C. 9-year-old child with ADHD and treatment-emergent tics
    D. 19-year-old with significant residual symptoms of ADHD
    E. All of the above

10. Which one of the following is not a dose-dependent side-effect of olanzapine?

A. Agranulocytosis
B. Akathisia
C. Galactorrhoea
D. Parkinsonism
E. Sedation

11. An anxious patient who has not responded to initial doses of clozapine titration wants to know about the dose-dependent side-effects of clozapine. Which one of the following is definitely not a dose-related risk?

A. Seizures
B. Hypersalivation
C. Sedation
D. Agranulocytosis
E. Anticholinergic effects

12. Acetyl cholinesterase and butyryl cholinesterase are two enzymes metabolizing acetylcholine. Which one of the following antidementia drugs has significant effects on both enzymes?

A. Galantamine
B. Rivastigmine
C. Ginkgo biloba
D. Memantine
E. Donepezil

13. A 66-year-old lady being treated for tremors by her neurologist develops insomnia, increased nocturnal myoclonus, and disruptive nightmares following the prescription of a particular medication. The most likely causative agent is

A. Bromocriptine
B. Levodopa
C. Propranolol
D. Pramipexole
E. Selegeline

14. A patient treated for severe Parkinson's disease develops troublesome psychotic symptoms attributed to levodopa. The neurologist is reluctant to reduce or stop levodopa given her deterioration in the past when this was attempted. The most appropriate drug to treat her psychotic symptoms is

A. Olanzapine
B. Risperidone
C. Quetiapine
D. Paliperidone
E. Bromocriptine

15. **Which one of the following drugs denatures the monoamine oxidase enzyme, rendering it ineffective to metabolize even low amounts of tyramine?**

    A. Selegiline
    B. Moclobemide
    C. Tranylcypromine
    D. Reboxetine
    E. None of the above

16. **Tyramine is present in certain food substances and can cause hypertensive crises if consumed by a patient on monoamine oxidase inhibitors. Choose the site of action of tyramine from the following options**

    A. Presynaptic storage vesicles
    B. Reuptake channels
    C. α_1 adrenergic receptors
    D. β adrenergic receptors
    E. α_2 autoreceptors

17. **Which one of the following antidepressants can block the neuronal uptake of tyramine and potentially reduce the risk of tyramine–MAOI interaction?**

    A. SSRIs
    B. Moclobemide
    C. L-tryptophan
    D. Tricyclic antidepressants
    E. Levothyroxine

18. **Which one of the following mood stabilizers can potentiate GABA transmission by increasing GABA release, reducing GABA metabolism, and increasing GABA receptor density?**

    A. Lithium
    B. Carbamazepine
    C. Lamotrigine
    D. Valproate
    E. Vigabatrin

19. **Which one of the following benzodiazepines has partial agonistic action at some receptors, leading to fewer withdrawal symptoms?**

    A. Diazepam
    B. Triazolam
    C. Lorazepam
    D. Clonazepam
    E. Chlordiazepoxide

20. **A patient presents with recurrent episodes of feeling detached and unreal. A pharmacological agent that can worsen the above symptoms is**

    A. Clozapine
    B. Caffeine
    C. Lamotrigine
    D. Clonazepam
    E. Valproate

21. **A 64-year-old man with schizophrenia is being treated for cirrhotic liver. Unfortunately, he develops a relapse of psychotic symptoms and needs a change in his antipsychotic prescription. The safest option with regard to his hepatic status is**

    A. Amisulpride
    B. Olanzapine
    C. Clozapine
    D. Risperidone
    E. Chlorpromazine

22. **The mechanism of action of St John's wort is**

    A. Serotonin antagonism
    B. Norepinephrine agonism
    C. MAO inhibition
    D. Multiple reuptake inhibition
    E. Membrane stabilization

23. **Which one of the following acts via opiate receptors and could be a potential agent to prevent relapse of alcohol use?**

    A. Naloxone
    B. Acamprosate
    C. Disulfiram
    D. Naltrexone
    E. Bupropion

24. **A 44-year-old man with bipolar disorder treated with lithium develops chronic back pain. His GP wants to prescribe a NSAID analgesic and asks you to choose a NSAID with the least potential to interact with lithium. You will choose**

    A. Ibuprofen
    B. Diclofenac
    C. Aspirin
    D. Ketorolac
    E. Indomethacin

25. **Stimulants are useful in ADHD. The symptom that best responds to stimulants is**

   A. Insomnia
   B. Hyperactivity
   C. Inattention
   D. Motor tics
   E. Conduct disturbance

26. **Atomoxetine is useful in children with ADHD. The mechanism of action is by**

   A. Norepinephrine reuptake inhibition
   B. Serotonin potentiation
   C. GABA potentiation
   D. Membrane stabilization
   E. Acetylcholine synthesis

27. **A 30-year-old known heroin user is brought to A&E after an overdose of heroin, with a GCS of 3, a respiratory rate of four breaths per minute, and pinpoint pupils. On administration of naloxone he develops running nose, diarrhoea and profuse sweating, and multiple joint aches. The most likely explanation is**

   A. Residual symptoms of toxicity
   B. Allergic reaction to naloxone
   C. Effect of coadministered cocaine
   D. Precipitated opioid withdrawal
   E. None of the above

28. **A 30-year-old known heroin user develops opioid intoxication which reverses on administration of naloxone. He takes a self-discharge against medical advice. He was brought back within a few hours of this self-discharge with signs suggestive of opioid intoxication, but without any history of additional opioid intake. The most likely explanation is**

   A. Inappropriate dose of naloxone
   B. Inappropriate route of administration of naloxone
   C. Short half-life of naloxone
   D. Reduced opioid tolerance on administering naloxone
   E. None of the above

29. **Naloxone can be life-saving in cases of opioid toxicity. The commonest route of administration of naloxone for this purpose is**

   A. Subcutaneous
   B. Intramuscular
   C. Transtracheal
   D. Intrathecal
   E. Intravenous

30. **Lofexidine is useful in managing symptoms of opiate withdrawal. The mechanism of action of lofexidine is by**
    A. Agonism of α_2 autoreceptors
    B. Direct opioid antagonism
    C. Partial opioid agonism
    D. Direct dopamine blockade
    E. Spinal opiate receptor blockade

31. **Fluoxetine increases the clinical efficacy of clozapine through which of the following pharmacokinetic mechanism?**
    A. Increased plasma protein binding
    B. Increased intestinal absorption
    C. Inhibition of hepatic metabolism
    D. Reduced renal clearance
    E. Improved blood–brain barrier penetration

32. **Tyramine can produce the 'cheese reaction' in patients taking MAO inhibitors. Which one of the following is true with respect to the moclobemide–tyramine interaction?**
    A. Moclobemide does not cause cheese reaction with tyramine
    B. Moclobemide causes cheese reaction at the same frequency as phenelzine
    C. Moclobemide does not act on the same enzyme that metabolizes tyramine
    D. Large consumption of tyramine can produce the cheese reaction with moclobemide
    E. All of the above

33. **Which one of the following is a partial opioid agonist with a low intrinsic activity?**
    A. Naloxone
    B. Naltrexone
    C. Methadone
    D. Buprenorphine
    E. None of the above

34. **A 12-year-old child treated for ADHD with stimulants develops tics, which persist even on withdrawal of stimulants. Which of the following offers a potential to treat both tics and ADHD symptoms simultaneously?**
    A. Clonidine
    B. Lofexidine
    C. Bromocriptine
    D. Atomoxetine
    E. Risperidone

35. **A 40-year-old male develops impotence secondary to antidepressant therapy. After trying various options, you are considering sildenafil. The mechanism of action of sildenafil is by**

   A. Phosphodiesterase inhibition
   B. Acetylcholine stimulation
   C. Increasing nitric oxide production
   D. Blockade of sympathetic discharge
   E. None of the above

36. **Buspirone is an anxiolytic with no immediate effect on acute administration, unlike diazepam. This is due to**

   A. Short half-life of buspirone
   B. Longer time required to achieve steady state
   C. Buspirone follows first-order kinetics
   D. Buspirone is a GABA partial agonist
   E. Buspirone acts via the serotonin system

37. **Most diuretics interact with lithium to produce significant changes in plasma lithium levels. Which one of the following diuretics is useful in treating polyuria, a common side-effect of lithium?**

   A. Amiloride
   B. Triamterene
   C. Chlorthiazide
   D. Frusemide
   E. None of the above

38. **A 30-year-old woman was diagnosed with paranoid schizophrenia. She has been hospitalized and is prescribed antipsychotics. Which one of the following treatment-emergent conditions is known to be associated with the risk of suicide?**

   A. Akathisia
   B. Anticholinergic symptoms
   C. Dystonia of the laryngeal muscles
   D. Neuroleptic malignant syndrome
   E. Tardive dyskinesia

39. **For typical neuroleptics, the antipsychotic effect on positive psychotic symptoms is strongly correlated with**

   A. D2 occupancy
   B. Half-life
   C. D4 occupancy
   D. 5-HT antagonism
   E. None of the above

40. **Memantine is an antidementia drug licensed for moderately severe Alzheimer's dementia. The mechanism by which memantine acts is**

    A. Inhibition of NMDA receptor
    B. Inhibition of calcium ion channels
    C. Stimulation of GABA output
    D. Stimulation of glutamate release
    E. Mimicking the effects of acetylcholine

41. **Phenytoin and lithium are said to have narrow therapeutic indices. The term therapeutic index refers to**

    A. Ratio between median toxic and median effective dose
    B. Rate of production of toxic effects at a constant dose
    C. Duration of persistence of toxic effects after the onset
    D. Proportion of patients who experience a specific side-effect
    E. None of the above

42. **The lower incidence of extrapyramidal side-effects due to clozapine compared to haloperidol is possibly related to**

    A. Duration of D2 receptor occupancy
    B. Glutamate blockade
    C. GABA release at basal ganglia
    D. Intrinsic partial agonistic activity at the D2 receptor
    E. All of the above

43. **The volume of distribution of a drug depends on all of the following except**

    A. Protein binding
    B. Lipid solubility
    C. Tissue binding
    D. Half-life
    E. None of the above

44. **Drug A is an anticonvulsant, metabolized to inactive metabolites by the CYP450 system. Drug B, which induces CYP450, is expected to produce which one of the following if coadministered with drug A?**

    A. Reduced concentration of inactive metabolites
    B. Reduced efficacy of drug A
    C. Increased metabolism of drug A resulting in increased efficacy
    D. Increased concentration of drug A in plasma
    E. None of the above

45. **Glucuronyl transferase acts on an antidepressant drug A and converts it into a more water-soluble component with less potency but a higher concentration in bile. This process is called**
    A. Conjugation
    B. Oxidation
    C. Saponification
    D. Depolarization
    E. Enzyme induction

46. **Metabolism of psychotropic drugs include phase 1 and phase 2 reactions. All of the following are phase 2 reactions except**
    A. Glucuronidation
    B. Methylation
    C. Oxidation
    D. N acetylation
    E. Sulfation

47. **Breastfeeding is contraindicated when certain psychotropics are administered. The characteristic features of such psychotropics that are secreted in breast milk include all except**
    A. High lipid solubility
    B. High degree of ionization
    C. Poor protein binding
    D. Low acidic property
    E. All of the above

48. **A 25-year-old postgraduate student is suffering from initial insomnia during his final year of study. He is asking for a hypnotic that will cause least disturbance to his sleep architecture. The best choice is**
    A. Diazepam
    B. Chloral hydrate
    C. Zolpidem
    D. Promethiazine
    E. Temazepam

49. **Selegiline is used as an antiparkinsonian agent. Its mechanism of action is**
    A. Dopamine receptor agonism
    B. Increased dopamine synthesis
    C. COMT inhibition
    D. MAO-A inhibition
    E. MAO-B inhibition

50. Which of the following antidepressants is most selectively serotonergic?

A. Fluoxetine
B. Paroxetine
C. Citalopram
D. Clomipramine
E. Venlafaxine

51. Which one of the following antipsychotics is strongly implicated in deaths due to QTc prolongation?

A. Quetiapine
B. Olanzapine
C. Pimozide
D. Risperidone
E. Aripiprazole

52. Which one of the following anticonvulsants follows zero-order kinetics on dose increase within therapeutic range?

A. Gabapentin
B. Phenytoin
C. Ethosuximide
D. Valproate
E. Lamotrigine

53. A patient suffering from gastritis is prescribed several psychotropic medications. She wants to know which part of her body will absorb most of these orally administered drugs. The correct answer is

A. Oral mucosa
B. Large intestine
C. Oesophagus
D. Stomach
E. Small intestine

54. A patient started on antidepressant treatment for a first episode of depression stopped the medication abruptly after an initial response. Which one of the following medications, if prescribed, has the highest chance of causing the most troublesome discontinuation reaction?

A. Mirtazapine
B. Mianserin
C. Fluoxetine
D. Paroxetine
E. Moclobemide

55. A patient started on paroxetine after the first episode of depression stopped the medication abruptly following an initial response. Apart from short half-life, higher incidence of discontinuation reaction following paroxetine is attributed to

    A. Cholinergic rebound
    B. Poor plasma protein binding
    C. High blood–brain barrier penetration
    D. Higher addictive potential
    E. None of the above

56. The tricyclic antidepressant which is most lethal on overdose is

    A. Dosulepin
    B. Imipramine
    C. Lofepramine
    D. Clomipramine
    E. Nortriptyline

57. A patient develops neuroleptic malignant syndrome secondary to antipsychotic prescription. Which one of the following properties of antipsychotics predicts a lower risk of producing neuroleptic malignant syndrome?

    A. High anticholinergic property
    B. High sedative effect
    C. Strong dopamine blockade
    D. α adrenergic blockade
    E. High potency

58. Which one of the following agents produces dysphoria, myoclonus, flu-like symptoms, ataxia, hyperacusis, and anxiety on withdrawal?

    A. Opioids
    B. Benzodiazepines
    C. Cannabis
    D. Procyclidine
    E. Amphetamines

59. Among antipsychotic agents, a high anticholinergic effect is noted for which one of the following pairs?

    A. Chlorpromazine and haloperidol
    B. Thioridazine and chlorpromazine
    C. Thioridazine and haloperidol
    D. Chlorpromazine and risperidone
    E. Risperidone and paliperidone

60. Severe perspiration unrelated to ambient temperature is a side-effect associated with the prescription of

A. SSRIs
B. Venlafaxine
C. TCAs
D. All of the above
E. None of the above

61. A 55-year-old patient with late-onset schizophrenia develops dystonia on administration of antipsychotics. He is prescribed anticholinergic medications for this side-effect. Which one of the following anticholinergic drugs is most stimulating in its properties?

A. Trihexyphenidyl
B. Procyclidine
C. Benztropine
D. Biperiden
E. Orphenadrine

62. A 55-year-old patient with late-onset schizophrenia develops dystonia on administration of antipsychotics. He is prescribed anticholinergic medications for this side-effect. Which one of the following anticholinergic drugs has the least abuse potential due to a relative lack of stimulating properties?

A. Trihexyphenidyl
B. Procyclidine
C. Benztropine
D. Biperiden
E. Orphenadrine

63. A 55-year-old patient with late-onset schizophrenia develops dystonia on administration of antipsychotics. He is prescribed trihexyphenidyl for this side-effect. Which one of the following properties makes this drug most stimulating of all anticholinergics?

A. Dopamine agonistic effect
B. Nicotinic stimulation
C. Endorphin release
D. Stimulation of cannabinoid receptors
E. None of the above

64. All of the following measures help to reduce postural tremors induced by lithium therapy except

A. Reducing caffeine intake
B. Using propranolol
C. Administering lithium at bed time
D. Dose reduction
E. Using procyclidine

65. **The half-life of donepezil in an elderly patient with dementia is around**

    A. 70 hours
    B. 24 hours
    C. 12 hours
    D. 6 hours
    E. 3 hours

66. **A patient taking disulfiram to support abstinence from alcohol decides to yield to his temptation and starts drinking but only a day after stopping disulfiram. Which one of the following is correct in this scenario?**

    A. Disulfiram irreversibly damages alcohol dehydrogenase.
    B. Disulfiram has a half-life of around 100 hours.
    C. Severity of the interaction does not depend on the dose of either agent.
    D. Disulfiram competitively inhibits aldehyde dehydrogenase.
    E. None of the above.

67. **Smoking can reduce extrapyramidal side-effects caused by antipsychotics through**

    A. Induction of hepatic metabolism of antipsychotics
    B. Increased renal elimination of antipsychotics
    C. Intestinal ischaemia reducing drug absorption
    D. Effect of nicotine on skeletal muscles
    E. None of the above

68. **Acamprosate is used in the management of alcohol dependence. Which of the following is correct?**

    A. Acamprosate must be started preferably 2 weeks before the deadline to stop drinking.
    B. Acamprosate is started only after abstinence is achieved.
    C. Acamprosate has no demonstrable effect on craving.
    D. Consuming alcohol when taking acamprosate will produce fatal toxicity.
    E. Acamprosate increases levels of disulfiram to a toxic range.

69. **The most common reason for using dantrolene sodium in psychiatric patients is**

    A. Serotonin syndrome
    B. Catatonia
    C. Neuroleptic malignant syndrome
    D. Dystonia
    E. Chorea

70. **Which of the following is correctly paired?**

    A. Pimozide: phenothiazine
    B. Chlorpromazine: diphenyl butyl piperidine
    C. Trifluperazine: aliphatic phenothiazine
    D. Thioridazine: dibenzoxapine
    E. Haloperidol: butyrophenone

71. **The most prominent mechanism of action of lamotrigine is**
    A. Calcium channel blockade
    B. Voltage-sensitive sodium channel blockade
    C. Glutamate antagonism
    D. Serotonin reuptake inhibition
    E. GABA potentiation

72. **The ECG changes produced by long-term lithium therapy mimic which one of the following electrolyte disturbances?**
    A. Hyperkalaemia
    B. Hypokalaemia
    C. Hypocalcaemia
    D. Hypercalcaemia
    E. Hyperuricaemia

73. **A 34-year-old lady with bipolar disorder responds well to lamotrigine. She develops a minor maculopapular rash 6 months after the onset of treatment. The most appropriate line of action is**
    A. Discontinue lamotrigine
    B. Persevere with lamotrigine as the rash is only minor
    C. This is very common and needs antihistaminic prescription
    D. Refer to dermatology but continue lamotrigine
    E. Reassure the patient and reduce the dose

74. **ECT is widely used to treat resistant and psychotic depression. Which of the following statements is correct with respect to the clinical use of ECT?**
    A. Seizure threshold varies widely among different individuals.
    B. Seizure threshold is fixed for each individual once the treatment is started.
    C. No correlation exist between electrical dose and amnesia.
    D. Incidence of cognitive disturbance is irrespective of the weekly frequency of administration.
    E. None of the above.

75. **Which one of the following antidepressants resembles amphetamine in chemical structure?**
    A. Buspirone
    B. Bupropion
    C. Imipramine
    D. Nortriptyline
    E. Duloxetine

76. Which of the following antidepressants is used by urologists for patients with incontinence?

    A. Citalopram
    B. Nortriptyline
    C. Paroxetine
    D. Duloxetine
    E. Venlafaxine

77. Which one of the following can increase plasma levels of lamotrigine?

    A. Lorazepam
    B. Chlorpromazine
    C. Valproate
    D. Carbamazepine
    E. Zopiclone

78. One of your regular out-patients with recurrent depression was recently started on a medication but comes back with aggravated psoriatic skin lesions. The most probable offending agent is

    A. Lithium
    B. Valproate
    C. Olanzapine
    D. Zopiclone
    E. Chlorpromazine

79. A 34-year-old man taking lithium twice daily experiences side-effects. Your consultant has advised him to take it once daily to reduce the side-effect. Which one of the following side-effects may respond to this intervention?

    A. Fine tremors
    B. Lethargy
    C. Polyuria
    D. Hypothyroidism
    E. Gastrointestinal distress

80. An intoxicated patient needs prescription for alcohol withdrawal. He is known to have cirrhosis with ascites. The benzodiazepine of choice is

    A. Diazepam
    B. Chlordiazepoxide
    C. Alprazolam
    D. Midazolam
    E. Oxazepam

81. Regular, long-term prescription of anticholinergics increases the risk of

    A. Akathisia
    B. Dytonia
    C. Parkinsonism
    D. Tardive dyskinesia
    E. Torticollis

82. **Select one drug associated with gastrointestinal bleeding**
    A. Benzodiazepines
    B. SSRIs
    C. MAOIs
    D. Methadone
    E. Bupropion

83. **Which of the following is a partial agonist at nicotinic acetylcholine receptors that can be used to promote smoking cessation?**
    A. Varenicline
    B. Bupropion
    C. Ticarcilline
    D. Dosulepin
    E. Gallantamine

84. **A 48-year-old man taking multiple drugs for hypertension, diabetes, and bipolar disorder presents with disabling impotence. Which of the following drugs that he might be using is not associated with sexual dysfunction?**
    A. Atenolol
    B. Fluphenazine
    C. Glibenclamide
    D. Thiazide diuretics
    E. α_1-blocker

85. **A 40-year-old man with chronic dysthymia also suffers from impotence unrelated to his depression. His GP prescribes him a medication to be used prior to the sexual act, as and when required. Which of the following describes the most likely mechanism of action of the prescribed drug?**
    A. Prostaglandin precursor
    B. Selective phosphodiesterase type 5 inhibition
    C. Selective serotonin uptake inhibition
    D. Dopamine agonist
    E. α adrenoceptor blockade

86. **Which of the following opioids produces metabolites with clinically useful analgesic activity?**
    A. Naloxone
    B. Nomifensine
    C. Propoxyphene
    D. Codeine
    E. Naltrexone

87. **The mechanism of action of opioids in producing an analgesic effect is**

    A. Blockade of sodium channels on the neuronal membrane (membrane stabilization)
    B. Increased production of cAMP in a neurone
    C. Reduction in intracellular calcium in a neurone
    D. Stimulation of Gs–protein-coupled receptors in the neurone
    E. Direct action on nuclear transcription factors

88. **Methylxanthines produce stimulation of the CNS via their action on which of the following receptors?**

    A. NMDA receptors
    B. Adenosine receptors
    C. Nicotinic receptors
    D. GABA receptors
    E. Cholinergic muscarinic receptors

89. **Which of the following medications used for Parkinson's disease is correctly paired with its side-effect?**

    A. Levodopa–hypoglycaemia
    B. Bromocriptine–hyperprolactinaemia
    C. Amantadine–livedo reticularis
    D. Tolcapone–gouty arthritis
    E. Bromocriptine–aplastic anaemia

90. **Which of the following agents acts through glial/ neuronal GABA reuptake inhibition?**

    A. Zopiclone
    B. Vigabatrin
    C. Topiramate
    D. Tiagabine
    E. Gabapentin

91. **Which of the following neuropharmacological agents is described as a melatonergic antidepressant?**

    A. Agomelatine
    B. L-tryptophan
    C. Melatonin
    D. Modafinil
    E. Ropinirole

92. **Which of the following medications can be used to treat narcolepsy and associated sleep disorders?**

    A. Buprenorphine
    B. Fluoxetine
    C. Imipramine
    D. Modafinil
    E. Naloxone

93. Which of the following drugs has some evidence for the treatment of resistant depression as an augmenting agent to SSRIs?

    A. Atenolol
    B. Labetolol
    C. Pentazocine
    D. Pindolol
    E. Tramadol

94. The half-life of atomoxetine in most individuals is

    A. 2 weeks
    B. 24 hours
    C. 36 hours
    D. 5 days
    E. 5 hours

95. Which of the following is considered to be the safest of all MAO-A inhibitors when used in combination with other antidepressants to treat depression?

    A. Isocarboxazid
    B. Isoniazid
    C. Phenelzine
    D. Selegiline
    E. Tranylcypromine

1.A. The dose at which side-effects develop is often determined at phase 1 of clinical trials. The pathway that a drug must follow before approval and marketing starts with animal studies, where the molecule is demonstrated to have specific actions. These extensive, preclinical animal studies must be carried out on at least two different animal species. Mutagenicity, carcinogenicity, and organ system toxicity are studies at this phase. A new drug under investigation then enters human trials. The first phase consists of determining if the drug is safe on human subjects. It is administered to a small group of volunteers and safety, tolerability, and pharmacokinetics of the drug are ascertained. In phase 2, effectiveness in comparison to placebo is studied in hundreds of patients with the target disease to see if it works at all against the disease. In phase 3, the drug undergoes extensive double-blind, randomized controlled trials to determine how well it works and what are the common side-effects. Phase 4 takes place if all the previous phases are successfully crossed—the drug undergoes the approval process by regulatory bodies and postmarketing surveillance ensues. Less common side-effects, which sometimes could lead to a drug's withdrawal, can be picked up when large-scale prescribing takes place during postmarketing surveillance.

Sadock BJ and Sadock VA. *Kaplan and Sadock's Comprehensive Textbook of Psychiatry*, 8th edn. Lippincott Williams and Wilkins, 2004. p. 2708.

2.C. Potency of a drug with receptor-binding action refers to the amount of the drug needed to produce a particular effect compared to another standard drug with similar receptor profile ('vigour'). Affinity refers to the ability of the drug to bind to its appropriate receptor ('affection'). Efficacy refers to how well the drug produces the expected response, that is the maximum clinical response produced by a drug ('productivity'). Efficacy depends on affinity, potency, duration of receptor action in some cases, and kinetic properties such as half-life, among other factors. Haloperidol is more potent than chlorpromazine as approximately 5 mg of haloperidol is required to achieve the same effect as 100 mg of chlorpromazine. These drugs, however, are equal in the maximal clinical response achievable using them, that is equally efficacious but not equipotent.

Sadock BJ and Sadock VA. *Kaplan and Sadock's Synopsis of Psychiatry: Behavioral Sciences/Clinical Psychiatry*, 10th edn. Lippincott Williams and Wilkins, 2007, p. 985.

3.E. After oral administration, a drug may be incompletely absorbed. This is mainly due to lack of absorption from the intestine related to the presence of inhibitory factors such as food or gastric acid, or to changes in intestinal motility; for example having diarrhoea or vomiting can affect drug absorption. Inherent properties of certain drugs can also affect their absorption, for example highly hydrophilic drugs cannot cross the lipid cell membrane, while highly lipophilic drugs will struggle to cross the water layer in extracellular space. Presence of reverse transporters, such as P-glycoprotein, can affect drug absorption. P-glycoprotein pumps certain drug molecules actively out into the gut lumen from gut cells. Inhibition of P-glycoprotein and gut wall metabolism, for example by grapefruit juice, can increase absorption of certain (mostly non-psychotropic) medications.

Sadock BJ and Sadock VA. *Kaplan and Sadock's Comprehensive Textbook of Psychiatry*, 8th edn. Lippincott Williams and Wilkins, 2004, p. 2700.

4. D. The blood–brain barrier poses a special challenge to the transit of drug molecules into the brain, which is very important to ensure the activity of most psychotropics. The blood–brain barrier is a structural and functional barrier comprised of capillary endothelium of brain, which possesses tight junctions, acting in unison as a single sheet or membrane. These junctions are disrupted when meningitis or other inflammation affects the structure. The ability of a drug to pass the blood–brain barrier depends on its molecular size, lipid solubility, and ionic status. Unionized molecules that are freely available and less protein bound are transported across the barrier easily. In general, the higher the lipid water partition coefficient, the greater the ability to cross the barrier. Exceptionally, there are a few molecules that pass the barrier effectively in spite of having a low lipid–water partition coefficient. These have specific carrier mechanisms, for example amino acid transport system (this is stereo specific, so that L amino acids but not D amino acids are easily transferred). L-dopa and valproate have specific carrier mechanisms. Some areas of brain lack this barrier—subfornical organ, area postrema, and median eminence. These circumventricular organs allow transfer of many compounds from blood to brain. This may have a survival benefit as certain toxic substances stimulate the area postrema and induce nausea and vomiting.

Johnstone E et al., eds. *Companion to Psychiatric Studies*, 7th edn. Churchill Livingstone, 2004, p. 38.

5. A. Pharmacokinetic changes in old age are pertinent when considering initiation, dosing, and coadministration of medications in the elderly. In general, the ability to absorb an orally administered medication is not greatly affected, but elderly patients have less body fat, and so lipid-soluble drugs may be distributed to brain tissue more avidly. However, this effect is not universal for all drugs. Protein binding and hepatic metabolism are reduced in elderly people, especially when malnourished. Renal function invariably drops with age. Note that this question is non-specific with respect to the prescribed drug.

Gelder MG et al., eds. *New Oxford Textbook of Psychiatry*. Oxford University Press, 2000, p. 1278.

6. D. Pindolol is a partial agonist at β-receptor sites. In addition, it is a 5-HT$_{1A}$ antagonist and has been studied as an augmenting agent with antidepressants. The final common pathway of action of most psychotropics is interference with neurotransmitter function. In general, neurotransmitters are released from a presynaptic neurone, occupy a receptor in a postsynaptic neurone, and bring about a change in the activity of the postsynaptic neurone. If a drug acts in a similar fashion to a neurotransmitter and brings about a similar change in the postsynaptic neurone, then it is called an agonist. This is often due to the intrinsic activity of the drug molecule on the specific receptors. Certain drugs occupy the receptors and do not have any intrinsic activity; they simply stop the neurotransmitter from carrying out its routine function. These drugs are called antagonists for the particular receptor. Certain other drugs have a degree of intrinsic activity; thus, when there is no indigenous neurotransmitter in the vicinity, they can produce a degree of effect similar to the neurotransmitter but if these molecules are allowed to compete with the indigenous neurotransmitters, this becomes counter productive. They block the full action that could be provided by the neurotransmitter. Hence, these are called partial agonists. Propranalol is a β-agonist with both β1- and β2-antagonistic properties. Olanzapine is predominantly a serotonin (5-HT$_{2A}$) and dopamine antagonist (D2). Carbamazepine is a membrane-stabilizing agent while the mechanism of action of lithium is thought to be mediated via the second messenger inositol system. The anxiolytic buspirone is a partial agonist at 5-HT$_{1A}$ autoreceptors. Aripiprazole is also a partial agonist at dopamine receptors.

Oliver JS, Cryan JF, Burrows GD et al. Pindolol augmentation of antidepressants: a review and rationale. *Australian and New Zealand Journal of Psychiatry* 2000; **34**: 71–79.

7. C. Amoxicillin is largely cleared through the kidneys and does not interfere with clozapine metabolism. Clozapine undergoes hepatic metabolism via CYP1A2, CYP3A4, and CYP2D6. Ciprofloxacin and other fluoroquinolone antibiotics can inhibit CYP1A2 and affect clozapine levels. Smoking induces CYP1A2 and quitting it will lead to a rebound inhibition effect on the enzyme appearing after 2 to 4 weeks. Byproducts of tobacco smoking, particularly the polycyclic aromatic hydrocarbons, are the major offenders in this regard. The metabolic inductive effects are not specific to tobacco smoking as they can also be expected from marijuana smoking. Erythromycin inhibits CYP3A4; this may lead to increase in clozapine levels. Caffeine has the opposite effect of smoking on clozapine metabolism. It inhibits CYP1A2 enzyme, leading to higher clozapine levels.

Worrel JA, Marken PA, Beckman SE et al. Atypical antipsychotic agents: A critical review. American Journal of Health-System Pharmacy 2000; **57**: 238–255.

8. A. Imipramine seems to be synergistic with ECT; it is shown to be more effective than SSRIs in preventing relapse following ECT in depressed patients (Lauritzen et al., 1996). Monoamine oxidase inhibitors have been shown to be more effective than tricyclics in atypical depressive disorders with biological features such as increased sleep and increased appetite. Though imipramine may not be as effective as MAOIs, it has been shown to be better than placebo in atypical depression. An often-quoted study that undertook head-to-head comparison of CBT and imipramine is the National Institute of Mental Health Depression Study (Elkin et al., 1989). In this study 16 weeks of CBT, imipramine, interpersonal therapy (IPT), and placebo were compared. Among the less-severely depressed patients, comparable proportions achieved remission in all three active treatment arms; but among the more-depressed patients, imipramine was superior to CBT in terms of remission rates achieved. Imipramine alters sleep structure considerably; it reduces REM (rapid eye movement) sleep and increases NREM (non-REM) sleep. All tricyclics are toxic in overdose; tertiary amines such as amitriptyline and imipramine produce longer-acting metabolites and have higher toxic potential than secondary amines.

Elkin I, Shea T, Watkins JT et al. National Institute of Mental Health treatment of depression collaborative research program. Archives of General Psychiatry 1989; **46**: 971–982.
Lauritzen L, Odgaard K, Clemmesen L et al. Relapse prevention by means of paroxetine in ECT-treated patients with major depression: a comparison with imipramine and placebo in medium-term continuation therapy. Acta Psychiatrica Scandinavica 1996; **94**: 241–251.
McGrath PJ, Stewart JW, Janal MN et al. A placebo-controlled study of fluoxetine versus imipramine in the acute treatment of atypical depression. American Journal of Psychiatry 2000; **157**: 344–350.

9. C. Treatment-emergent tics and dyskinesias are often self-limited over 7 to 10 days in children taking stimulants. In some cases, if the severity of tics necessitates a dose reduction, adjustments can be made in the medication dosage. In severe cases, atomoxetine could be prescribed after stopping stimulants. Methylphenidate may also worsen already existing tics in one-third of patients. In most of these cases tics are variable, depending on the plasma levels. They resolve immediately on clearance of the drug. In the rest, tics are triggered by the treatment and persist for several months. It is appropriate to continue treating an adult with residual, disabling symptoms of ADHD. Though stimulants can exacerbate psychosis, a family history of psychosis is not a contraindication. Family history of ADHD does not adversely influence stimulant prescription.

Taylor D et al., eds. The Maudsley Prescribing Guidelines, 9th edn. Informa Healthcare, 2007, p. 281.

10. A. Olanzapine can induce agranulocytosis, similar to clozapine albeit at much lower frequency. Atypicality of atypical antipsychotics does not exist as a dichotomous entity from typical drugs. At high doses, most atypical agents lose their atypicality and produce extrapyramidal symptoms and galactorrhoea. Large weight gains with increased appetite occur during the first 6 months of treatment, irrespective of the dose used. The risk of weight gain continues over time, probably reaching a peak after 9 months, after which it slows down but continues as long as one takes the drug. Weight gain is associated with increased total cholesterol. Olanzapine is also associated with dose-dependent sedation, though tolerance usually develops for this effect.

Tolosa-Vilella C et al. Olanzapine-induced agranulocytosis: a case report and review of the literature. *Progress in Neuro-psychopharmacology and Biological Psychiatry* 2002; **26**: 411–414.

11. D. Agranulocytosis is not dose dependent; it is idiosyncratic. A reduction in dose of clozapine cannot help a patient who has developed agranulocytosis. Clozapine-associated seizures are clearly dose related. When doses of clozapine below 300 mg/day are used, the seizure rate remains 1%; further doses between 300 and 600 mg/day increase the seizure rate to 2.7%, and doses above 600 mg/day have a rate of 4.4%. Slower dose titration, using a lower dose, and the addition of anticonvulsant agent such as valproic acid can reduce the frequency of seizures. Anticholinergic effects, such as tachycardia and constipation, may be dose dependent, and are often noted in overdoses. Similar to sialorrhoea, clozapine-related tachycardia is often seen in early phases of treatment, and tolerance develops in due course.

Taylor D et al., eds. *The Maudsley Prescribing Guidelines*, 9th edn. Informa Healthcare, 2007, pp. 71, 73, and 81.

12. B. Donepezil and galantamine are selective inhibitors of acetylcholinesterase enzyme. Rivastigmine affects both butyryl and acetyl cholinesterase. Galantamine also affects nicotinic receptors. However, these differences do not translate into significant clinical differences in efficacy or tolerability. Memantine is an N-methyl-D-aspartic acid (NMDA) antagonist and hence is thought to be a neuroprotective agent. Tacrine was one of the foremost anticholinesterases introduced but is no longer used due to hepatotoxic effects. Tacrine inhibits both acetyl and butyrylcholinesterases. Ginkgo biloba is widely used in Germany as a cognitive enhancer. Its mechanism of action is unclear.

Taylor D et al., eds. *The Maudsley Prescribing Guidelines*, 9th edn. Informa Healthcare, 2007, p. 415. Leonard BE. Pharmacotherapy in the treatment of Alzheimer's disease: an update. *World Psychiatry* 2004; **3**: 84–88.

13. B. Levodopa is used to treat symptoms of Parkinson's disease. Levodopa is associated with increase in libido; in some cases secondary mania is reported. It can cause disruptive nightmares and forced reminiscences. It is a stimulating medication and can produce initial insomnia and nocturnal myoclonus. It is also associated with belpharospasms. Bromocriptine and pramipexole are dopamine agonists while selegeline is a monoamine oxidase B (MAO-B) inhibitor used in treating Parkinson's disease.

Sadock BJ and Sadock VA. *Kaplan and Sadock's Comprehensive Textbook of Psychiatry*, 8th edn. Lippincott Williams and Wilkins, 2004, p. 410.

14. C.   Psychosis is common in patients with Parkinson's disease. This may be due to the use of dopaminergic medications such as levodopa or unrelated to the pathology of Parkinson's disease. Lewy body dementia can result in psychotic features and prominent parkinsonism, in which case antipsychotic treatment may be required. In such cases and in levodopa-induced psychosis, quetiapine has been used as the treatment of choice as it has a very low extrapyramidal side-effects profile. Clozapine is also equally useful and generally regarded as the gold standard. In Parkinson's disease-related psychosis even low doses of atypical antipsychotics can result in good efficacy.

Sadock BJ and Sadock VA. *Kaplan and Sadock's Comprehensive Textbook of Psychiatry*, 8th edn. Lippincott Williams and Wilkins, 2004, p. 411.

15. C.   Tyramine is predominantly metabolized by MAO-A enzyme present in gut wall and liver, apart from brain and other tissues. Drugs which irreversibly inhibit MAO-A affect tyramine metabolism. These include tranylcypromine and phenelzine. Drugs such as selegiline are irreversible MAO-B selective inhibitors; they do not have the same effect on tyramine as MAO-A inhibitors. Moclobemide is a reversible, somewhat competitive MAO-A selective inhibitor. Thus, when the relative amount of tyramine in the vicinity increases, the moclobemide molecule makes way for tyramine from the MAO-A enzyme site. Reboxetine is not an MAO inhibitor.

Sadock BJ and Sadock VA. *Kaplan and Sadock's Comprehensive Textbook of Psychiatry*, 8th edn. Lippincott Williams and Wilkins, 2004, p. 2855.

16. A.   Tyramine is a monoamine naturally occurring in many food substances. Generally, most ingested tyramine undergoes a complete breakdown in the periphery due to the action of MAO-A enzyme in gut mucosa and liver. When a patient is taking MAO-A inhibitor drugs, tyramine escapes such degradation and enters the brain through amino acid transport. It uses the norepinephrine reuptake channels, and gains entry to presynaptic neurones. Here, tyramine stimulates release of all bound monoamines, especially norepinephrine, leading to a hypertensive reaction. This is called the cheese reaction as tyramine is abundant in mature cheeses.

Sadock BJ and Sadock VA. *Kaplan and Sadock's Comprehensive Textbook of Psychiatry*, 8th edn. Lippincott Williams and Wilkins, 2004, p. 2860.

17. D.   As tyramine gains entry to presynaptic neurones via the norepinephrine transporter, blocking this reuptake transporter can prevent tyramine action, at least theoretically. Tricyclic antidepressants act via blockade of this transporter. Hence the incidence of cheese reaction due to tyramine is less in those who are on tricyclic antidepressants before the commencement of MAO-A inhibitors. However, such combination is not advisable as the potential to cause serotonin syndrome is very high. SSRIs and L-tryptophan can increase the risk of serotonin syndrome many fold when coprescribed with MAO-A inhibitors.

Sadock BJ and Sadock VA. *Kaplan and Sadock's Comprehensive Textbook of Psychiatry*, 8th edn. Lippincott Williams and Wilkins, 2004, p. 2965.
White K and Simpson G. Combined MAOI-tricyclic antidepressant treatment: a re-evaluation. *Journal of Clinical Psychopharmacology* 1981; **1**: 264–282.

18. D. The mechanism of action of lithium remains speculative. Valproate increases gamma-aminobutyric acid (GABA) release and reduces GABA metabolism. It increases neuronal responsiveness to GABA and also increases $GABA_B$ receptor density. Carbamazepine prolongs sodium channel inactivation, leading to a secondary increase in calcium channel inactivation. This is linked to reduced glutamatergic neurotransmission. Carbamazepine also has adenosine antagonistic properties. Lamotrigine acts via membrane stabilization while vigabatrin is a GABA transaminase inhibitor.

Sadock BJ and Sadock VA. *Kaplan and Sadock's Comprehensive Textbook of Psychiatry*, 8th edn. Lippincott Williams and Wilkins, 2004, p. 2757.

19. D. Clonazepam has partial agonistic action at certain benzodiazepine receptors, leading to fewer withdrawal symptoms. Clonazepam is a high-potency drug (0.25 mg clonazepam is equated to 5 mg diazepam); it is shown to be effective in panic disorder and social phobia (but is not recommended for long-term therapy). In bipolar type 1 disorder, clonazepam may result in a prolonged remission phase and reduced depressive relapses when used as an adjuvant to lithium or lamotrigine, respectively.

Haefely W *et al*. Novel anxiolytics that act as partial agonists at benzodiazepine receptors. *Trends in Pharmacological Science* 1990; **11**: 452–456.

20. D. Caffeine can worsen depersonalization. Experimental induction of depersonalization and derealization has been tried using caffeine. SSRIs are used in treating established cases of depersonalization disorder. However, paradoxically, some times initiation or discontinuation of SSRIs can produce depersonalization experiences. Lamotrigine and clonazepam are used in treating symptoms of depersonalization.

Medford N *et al*. Understanding and treating depersonalization disorder. *Advances in Psychiatric Treatment* 2005; **11**: 92–100.

21. A. Most psychotropic medications undergo hepatic metabolism. Notable exceptions are amisulpride, paliperidone, lithium, acamprosate, and gabapentin. These medications are largely renally excreted without much hepatic degradation. Hence in patients with hepatic failure, the antipsychotic of choice from the given list is amisulpride. Note that certain benzodiazepines, such as oxazepam, undergo glucuronide conjugation (phase 2 metabolism) reaction but no oxidation (phase 1 metabolism) in the liver. Oxazepam can be used in treating alcohol withdrawal in a patient with significantly low hepatic reserve.

Taylor D *et al*., eds. *The Maudsley Prescribing Guidelines*, 9th edn. Informa Healthcare, 2007, p. 404.

22. D. St John's wort has been shown to be an effective antidepressant in mild to moderate cases. It increases photosensitivity of skin but other adverse effects are limited. It is thought to act by inhibiting reuptake of multiple monoamines, including serotonin, norepinephrine, and dopamine. It also inhibits GABA and glutamate reuptake but the effects of these are unknown. It is a potent inducer of hepatic CYP450 enzymes, leading to a fall in plasma levels of carbamazepine, oral contraceptives, and warfarin if coprescribed.

Taylor D *et al*., eds. *The Maudsley Prescribing Guidelines*, 9th edn. Informa Healthcare, 2007, p. 244.

23. D. Opioid receptor antagonists are tested as adjuncts for the treatment of alcohol dependence. They can reduce alcohol craving and alcohol consumption. If naltrexone is used in maintaining abstinence, the number of relapses is reduced and the severity of relapses, if they occur, is considerably less. Naloxone is a parenterally administered opioid antagonist, used to reverse the effects of exogenously administered opioids. Acamprosate, bupropion, and disulfiram do not act via an opioid mechanism.

Taylor D *et al*., eds. *The Maudsley Prescribing Guidelines*, 9th edn. Informa Healthcare, 2007, p. 332.

24. C. Aspirin (and sulindac, to some extent) has comparatively lesser potential to interact with lithium compared to most other NSAIDs. NSAIDs can reduce renal lithium clearance via their effects on fluid balance. This can lead to renal toxicity if the coadministration is sufficiently long. Indometacin is suspected to be worse compared to other NSAIDs in this regard, though careful monitoring of lithium levels is warranted even with use of COX-2 inhibitors such as rofecoxib. Lithium excretion is decreased by medications such as thiazides, angiotensin-converting enzyme inhibitors, and, to a lesser extent, frusemide (furosemide). Lithium clearance is increased by other medications with diuretic effects such as acetazolamide, mannitol, and caffeine.

Reimann IW, Diener U, and Frölich JC. Indomethacin but not aspirin increases plasma lithium ion levels. *Archives of General Psychiatry* 1983; **40**: 283–286.

25. B. Stimulants such as methylphenidate are more effective in treating hyperactivity than inattention due to ADHD. Methylphenidate is available in two forms—immediate release and sustained release forms. The immediate release form starts to act within 20 to 60 minutes after administration and acts for up to 2 to 4 hours, while the sustained release form acts up to 12 hours, obviating the need for divided doses.

Taylor D *et al.*, eds. *The Maudsley Prescribing Guidelines*, 9th edn. Informa Healthcare, 2007, p. 281.

26. A. Atomoxetine is the first non-stimulant drug to be approved for ADHD. It has a tricyclic-like structure; it is classified as a phenylpropanolamine derivative. It acts through selective inhibition of the presynaptic norepinephrine transporter. It has a half-life of approximately 5 hours and is metabolized through the CYP2D6 pathway. Drugs such as fluoxetine, paroxetine or bupropion are CYP2D6 inhibitors and may raise atomoxetine levels. Atomoxetine is used for patients who find stimulants too activating or who experience other intolerable side-effects. Atomoxetine has been associated with cases of severe liver injury in a few patients. It must be avoided in patients taking MAOI.

Sadock BJ and Sadock VA. *Kaplan and Sadock's Synopsis of Psychiatry: Behavioral Sciences/Clinical Psychiatry*, 10th edn. Lippincott Williams and Wilkins, 2007, p. 1103.

27. D. Naloxone is an opioid antagonist. It can precipitate acute withdrawal when administered to patients who are actively taking opioid drugs. Symptoms of acute opioid withdrawal include a strong urge to seek the drug, feeling of temperature change, pain, and abdominal distress. Patient may also have confusion, drowsiness, vomiting, and diarrhoea. When opioid antagonists that act for a long duration, such as naltrexone, are prescribed to encourage abstinence and maintain remission in opioid users it is absolutely essential that the use of street drugs has been completely stopped for at least a period of 5 to 7 days. If not, acute withdrawal symptoms will be precipitated. Naloxone produces opioid antagonism that lasts less than 1 hour, whereas naltrexone-induced withdrawal can persist for more than 24 hours.

Sadock BJ and Sadock VA. *Kaplan and Sadock's Synopsis of Psychiatry: Behavioral Sciences/Clinical Psychiatry*, 10th edn. Lippincott Williams and Wilkins, 2007, p. 1076.

28. C. Naloxone produces opioid antagonism that lasts less than 1 hour, as its plasma half-life is between 1 and 2 hours. In opioid overdose, naloxone is administered intravenously and repeated at 2- to 3-minute intervals until the desired response is achieved. In order to maintain recovery in significant overdoses, it is often necessary to continue naloxone by infusion or repeated administration. As this has not happened in the patient described in this question, signs of intoxication have returned.

Gelder MG *et al.*, eds. *New Oxford Textbook of Psychiatry*. Oxford University Press, 2000, p. 1339.

29. E. Naloxone is commonly administered via intravenous injections in the UK. It can also be administered intramuscularly or via subcutaneous injections.

Wanger K, Brough L, Macmillan I et al. Intravenous vs. subcutaneous naloxone for out-of-hospital management of presumed opioid overdose. *Academic Emergency Medicine* 1998; **5**: 293–299.

30. A. Lofexidine is an analogue of clonidine, and licensed only in the UK for use in opiate detoxification. It is an α_2 adrenoceptor agonist, similar to clonidine but it causes significantly less hypotension. Action of lofexidine peaks at 3 hours and its elimination half-life is 12–15 hours. It is administered in divided doses to achieve the desired peak effect coincidental with the peak of withdrawal effects. It is used for 1 to 3 weeks in opiate detoxification, with or without substituting a tapering dose of prescribed opiates. α_2 agonism leads to increased autoreceptor activity and resultant reduction in sympathetic stimulation, which mediates the withdrawal symptoms when administration of opioids is suddenly stopped.

Gelder MG et al., eds. *New Oxford Textbook of Psychiatry*. Oxford University Press, 2000, p. 1340.

31. C. SSRIs, especially fluoxetine, inhibit CYP2D6 enzyme involved in the metabolism of clozapine. This results in an increase in clozapine levels, leading to additional therapeutic advantage. This combination strategy has been tried in patients whose psychotic symptoms are refractory to clozapine. Therapeutic use of this interaction should be considered only when compliance is assured, maximal dosing has been achieved, and despite this the serum level is below 350 ng/ml. It should be attempted cautiously and with regular monitoring of plasma levels. When adding an SSRI, the dose of clozapine should be reduced in anticipation of the likely rise in plasma concentrations—an approximately twofold dose reduction is suggested for fluoxetine and paroxetine.

Williams L, Newton G, Roberts K et al. Clozapine-resistant schizophrenia: a positive approach. *British Journal of Psychiatry* 2002; **181**: 184–187.

32. D. Moclobemide acts on the same MAO-A enzyme that metabolizes tyramine, but the effect of moclobemide on this enzyme is reversible, leading to a lesser propensity of moclobemide to cause the tyramine reaction. When an unusually large consumption of tyramine-containing products occurs, moclobemide can produce the cheese reaction similar to other MAO inhibitors. Due to the reversible and partly competitive nature of MAO-A blockade by moclobemide, normal activity of existing MAO-A returns within 16 to 48 hours of the last dose of moclobemide. Therefore, the dietary restrictions are less stringent, reducing the avoidance of foods with a high concentrations of tyramine to a period from 1 hour before to 2 hours after taking moclobemide. These foods must be avoided only for 3 days after the last dose of moclobemide, unlike other MAO inhibitors where several days of diet is needed even after withdrawing the medication.

Sadock BJ and Sadock VA. *Kaplan and Sadock's Synopsis of Psychiatry: Behavioral Sciences/Clinical Psychiatry*, 10th edn. Lippincott Williams and Wilkins, 2007, p. 1068.

33. D. Buprenorphine is a partial μ-opioid agonist. It has a slow onset of action and dissociates rather slowly from the μ-receptor. It has very poor oral bioavailability and so is administered sublingually. The half-life of buprenorphine is only 3 to 5 hours but its action is rather prolonged due to slow dissociation of the drug molecule from the receptor—this phase lasts for more than 24 hours. Due to its partial agonistic action, the propensity to cause respiratory depression is lower than that of heroin. When overdose occurs, naloxone must be given at a higher dose and in continuous infusion to reverse the toxicity.

Gelder MG et al., eds. *New Oxford Textbook of Psychiatry*. Oxford University Press, 2000, p. 1338.

34. A. Clonidine is a central α_2 agonist. As the α_2 receptor is an autoreceptor, which on stimulation reduces sympathetic output, clonidine acts as sympatholytic drug. It is useful in some patients with tics and in Tourette's syndrome. As many drug withdrawal states are mediated by sympathetic overdrive, clonidine can potentially be used in opioid, alcohol, or benzodiazepine withdrawal though this is not a licensed indication. In children with ADHD, clonidine can be used as a third-line agent after stimulants and atomoxetine. However, it is rarely used for pure ADHD symptoms; it is commonly used when ADHD is accompanied by motor tics. Clonidine can cause significant hypotension.

Tourette's Syndrome Study Group. Treatment of ADHD in children with tics. A randomized controlled trial. *Neurology* 2002; **58**: 527–536.

35. A. Sexual arousal in a man results in the release of nitric oxide (NO) in vascular endothelium, mediated by autonomic nervous signals. NO acts as a second messenger and stimulates the synthesis of cyclic guanosine monophosphate (cGMP). This initiates a chain reaction, which results in corpus cavernosal relaxation and an increase in blood flow into the penis. This is followed by erection. Once produced, cGMP is cleared by the action of an intracellular enzyme called phosphodiesterase-5 (PDE-5). When PDE-5 is inhibited, the concentration of cGMP increases intracellularly, leading to prolonged tumescence and turgidity of the penis. Hence sexual arousal is required for PDE-5 inhibitors to have an effect on performance. Sildenafil acts as a PDE-5 inhibitor, allowing an increase in cGMP and enhancing the vasodilatory effects of NO. Hence it is sometimes referred to as an NO enhancer, but it does not have a direct effect on NO synthesis.

Sadock BJ and Sadock VA. *Kaplan and Sadock's Synopsis of Psychiatry: Behavioral Sciences/Clinical Psychiatry*, 10th edn. Lippincott Williams and Wilkins, 2007, p. 1078.

36. E. Buspirone is an azapirone which, by partial agonistic action on the 5-HT$_{1A}$ receptor, suppresses activity in presynaptic serotonergic neurones. This in turn reduces the serotonin activity, leading to down-regulation of various 5-HT receptors. This is related to anxiolytic activity but with no hypnotic effect. Though buspirone is equieffective to diazepam, patients taking buspirone improve more slowly. This is related to the inherent mode of action, which depends on receptor down-regulation rather than producing a direct receptor action. Patients who are switched from benzodiazepines to buspirone do not do as well as those without previous exposure to benzodiazepines.

Gelder MG et al., eds. *New Oxford Textbook of Psychiatry.* Oxford University Press, 2000, p. 1289.

37. A. Amiloride is useful in some cases of lithium-induced polyuria. Polyuria is the most common adverse effect of lithium, occurring in 25% of patients. This polyuria is related to the antagonistic effects of lithium on antidiuretic hormone, leading to diuresis. Conservative management includes fluid replacement, decreasing the dosage of lithium, and single daily dosing of lithium. Potassium-sparing diuretics, such as triamterene and amiloride, or thiazide diuretics are also useful. Unlike thiazides and frusemide, amiloride does not reduce lithium clearance; instead it may increase lithium excretion.

Sadock BJ and Sadock VA. *Kaplan and Sadock's Synopsis of Psychiatry: Behavioral Sciences/Clinical Psychiatry*, 10th edn. Lippincott Williams and Wilkins, 2007, p. 1059.

38. A. Akathisia is the commonest movement disorder associated with antipsychotic prescription. It is more commonly acute, with onset within 48 to 96 hours of administration of the antipsychotics. It is unclear whether akathisia results from dopamine antagonism or dysfunction of other neurotransmitters such as serotonin, acetyl choline, and norepinephrine. Akathisia is often mistaken for anxiety or worsening of psychotic agitation. Akathisia can vary in severity over time, making assessment difficult. Akathisia is associated with suicidality, absconsion, aggression, and non-compliance. Tardive dyskinesia develops late in the course of antipsychotic treatment and as such is not associated with absconsion from in-patient units, as more often than not the patients do not recognize having troublesome movement disorders. Neuroleptic malignant syndrome and laryngeal dystonia are life-threatening syndromes, often requiring immediate medical attention.

Hansen L. A critical review of akathisia—and its possible association with suicidal behaviour. *Human Psychopharmacology* 2001; **16**: 495–505.

39. A. D2 occupancy in typical antipsychotics correlates with their antipsychotic efficacy and propensity to cause extrapyramidal side-effects. This was demonstrated in a landmark positron emission tomography (PET) study by Kapur *et al.*, where haloperidol produced therapeutic effect at around 65% occupancy; extrapyramidal side-effects occurred when the occupancy was around 78%. For atypicals, both 5-HT$_{2A}$ blockade and D2 occupancy are correlated with clinical efficacy. Clozapine and quetiapine occupy less than half of D2 receptors but still are efficacious as antipsychotics.

Jones MM and Pilowsky LS. Dopamine and antipsychotic drug action revisited. *British Journal of Psychiatry* 2002; **181**: 271.

40. A. Memantine has moderate affinity for the NMDA receptor and acts as a voltage-dependent and non-competitive antagonist. Calcium-mediated excitotoxicity could be due to overstimulation of NMDA receptors by glutamate. Memantine may protect cells against excess glutamate by partially blocking NMDA receptors associated with abnormal transmission of glutamate, while physiological transmission remains unaffected.

Johnstone E *et al.*, eds. *Companion to Psychiatric Studies*, 7th edn. Churchill Livingstone, 2004, p. 303.

41. A. Therapeutic index is a measure that relates the dose of a drug required to produce a desired effect to that which produces an undesired effect. In animal studies, the therapeutic index is usually defined as the ratio of the median toxic dose to the median effective dose for some therapeutically relevant effect. The therapeutic index of a drug in humans cannot be measured directly and the value itself does not have much clinical use; instead, drug trials often reveal a range of usually effective doses and a range of possibly toxic doses, from which a safe therapeutic range is determined, for example 1.0 to 1.2 for lithium which when exceeded results in toxic effects.

Sadock BJ and Sadock VA. *Kaplan and Sadock's Comprehensive Textbook of Psychiatry*, 8th edn. Lippincott Williams and Wilkins, 2004, p. 2685.

42. A.   Clozapine has a hit-and-run profile at D2 receptors. The occupancy is around 40% and the time course of occupancy is comparatively shorter than typical antipsychotics. Quetiapine has a similar mode of action to that of clozapine. Clozapine and quetiapine bind more loosely to D2 receptors than dopamine itself whereas haloperidol and risperidone bind to these receptors more tightly. It is suggested that antipsychotics with low binding affinity and fast dissociation rates, such as clozapine and quetiapine, are more responsive to endogenous changes in dopamine than those that bind more tightly and dissociate from the receptor more slowly. This is because baseline dopamine levels are interspersed with task- or stress-induced, several-fold increases in dopamine from normal physiological level.

Pani L, Pira L, and Marchese G. Antipsychotic efficacy: Relationship to optimal D2-receptor occupancy. *European Psychiatry* 2007; **22**: 267–275.

43. D.   Volume of distribution is a measure of the apparent space in the body available to contain an administered drug. It can be calculated as a ratio of the administered dose (intravenous) and plasma (or blood) concentration at time = 0, that is when administration occurred. Hence, the higher the plasma concentration, the lower the volume of distribution and vice versa. Volume of distribution can vastly exceed any physical volume in the body because it is an apparent, not an actual, volume necessary to contain a drug homogeneously at the concentration found in the plasma. Drugs with very high volumes of distribution have higher concentrations in extravascular tissue than in the vascular compartment, while those that are contained fully in the vascular compartment have a smaller volume of distribution limited by the volume of plasma component. The apparent volume of distribution depends on properties of the drug molecule, such as lipid solubility and protein binding. Tissue binding decreases the plasma concentration and makes the apparent volume larger. Plasma protein binding increases plasma concentration and makes the apparent volume smaller. Half-life is a secondary measurement calculated from the volume of distribution and clearance rates, but volume of distribution itself does not depend on half-life of a drug. If the rate of clearance is slower or the volume of distribution is more extensive, the half-life will be longer.

Sadock BJ and Sadock VA. *Kaplan and Sadock's Comprehensive Textbook of Psychiatry*, 8th edn. Lippincott Williams and Wilkins, 2004, p. 2702.

44. B.   The cytochrome P450 (CYP450) enzyme system is responsible for much of the phase 1 metabolism of drugs. Phase 1 metabolism includes oxidation, reduction, and hydrolysis, as a result of which a molecule (active or inactive) suitable for conjugation is produced. The phase 2 metabolism involves conjugation reactions such as glucuronidation, as a result of which polar compounds (mostly inactive), which are excretable in bile or urine, are formed. Induction and inhibition of the activity of the CYP450 system can result in various potential drug interactions. The most important enzymes in the CYP family involved in the metabolism of psychotropic drugs are CYP1A2, CYP2C9, CYP2C19, CYP2D6, and CYP3A4. CYP3A4 is responsible for the metabolism of more than 90% of psychotropic drugs that undergo hepatic biotransformation. In this question, if the CYP system is induced then the metabolic breakdown of drug A will be increased, producing more inactive metabolites. This will reduce the efficacy of drug A.

Chadwick B, Waller DG, and Edwards JG *et al.* Potentially hazardous drug interactions with psychotropics. *Advances in Psychiatric Treatment* 2005; **11**: 440–449.

45. A.   Conjugation refers to phase 2 metabolism of administered drugs. These take place after oxidation-type reactions in phase 1. Enzymes such as transferases carry out conjugation, which usually results in inactive metabolites (or, rarely, active compounds, e.g. morphine). It is not essential that a drug must undergo phase 1 metabolism in order to undergo phase 2 metabolism, for example oxazepam undergoes direct phase 2 reactions.

Cookson J et al., eds. Use of Drugs in Psychiatry: The Evidence from Psychopharmacology, 5th edn. Gaskell, 2002, p. 57.

46. C.   Oxidation is not a phase 2 reaction—it is a phase 1 reaction. Various types of phase 2 reactions include glucuronidation, acetylation, sulfation, and glutathione conjugation. Hydrolysis and hydroxylation are considered to be other phase 1 reactions.

Cookson J et al., eds. Use of Drugs in Psychiatry: The Evidence from Psychopharmacology, 5th edn. Gaskell, 2002, p. 57.

47. B.   Most prescribed drugs transfer into breast milk except very large molecules such as heparin and insulin, but the amount transferred is negligent for most drugs. The mechanism of transfer is passive diffusion through the lipid cell membrane of the lactating glands. Factors such as low plasma protein binding and high lipid solubility aid a drug in reaching high concentrations in breast milk. As milk is slightly more acidic than plasma, weakly basic drugs transfer more readily into breast milk, become ionized in the acid medium, and so get 'trapped'. Unionized molecules cross biological membranes more easily than charged particles (ions). If a breastfeeding mother must take psychotropics and the drug is a relatively safe one, it is recommended that the drug is taken 30–60 minutes after nursing and 3–4 hours before the next feed, if possible.

Cohen D. Psychotropic medication and breast feeding. Advances in Psychiatric Treatment 2005; **11**: 371–379.

48. C.   Zolpidem is a non-benzodiazepine hypnotic of the imidazopyridine class. It is rapidly absorbed and has a short elimination half-life (mean 2.5 hours). It decreases sleep-onset latency, reduces disruptive midnight awakenings but has less consistent effects on total sleep time. It does not affect the REM distribution and unlike benzodiazepines, which increase stage 2 NREM at the expense of deep sleep NREM, zolpidem does not increase stage 2. It is unclear if zolpidem produces clinically significant rebound as yet but dependence is thought to be low compared to other hypnotics.

Darcourt G, Pringuey D, Sallière D, and Lavoisy J. The safety and tolerability of zolpidem—an update. Journal of Psychopharmacology 1999; **13**: 81–93.

49. E.   Two types of monoamine oxidase have been recognized: monoamine oxidase A predominantly metabolizes norepinephrine and serotonin; monoamine oxidase B predominantly metabolizes dopamine. Selegiline is a selective inhibitor of monoamine oxidase B that retards the breakdown of dopamine and so it prolongs the antiparkinsonism effect of levodopa as an adjunctive therapy for patients with fluctuating response to levodopa. Some studies have found it to be effective for treating depression but only at very high doses at which selective MAO-B inhibition effect is taken over by non-specific inhibition.

Sadock BJ and Sadock VA. Kaplan and Sadock's Synopsis of Psychiatry: Behavioral Sciences/Clinical Psychiatry, 10th edn. Lippincott Williams and Wilkins, 2007, p. 1070.

50. C. Citalopram (and escitalopram) is the most selective inhibitor of serotonin reuptake, with negligible effects on the reuptake of other monoamines such as norepinephrine or dopamine. It does not have any clinically significant effect on histaminergic, GABAergic, or acetylcholinergic transmission. Paroxetine has clinically significant anticholinergic activity. Fluoxetine weakly inhibits norepinephrine reuptake and binds to 5-HT$_{2C}$ receptors. Sertraline weakly inhibits both norepinephrine and dopamine reuptake, without any additional clinical advantage.

Sadock BJ and Sadock VA. *Kaplan and Sadock's Synopsis of Psychiatry: Behavioral Sciences/Clinical Psychiatry*, 10th edn. Lippincott Williams and Wilkins, 2007, p. 1085.

51. C. Prolongation of the QT interval of the ECG is associated with the development of torsade de pointes, a ventricular arrhythmia that can cause syncope and may progress to ventricular fibrillation and sudden death. The average QTc interval is approximately 400 ms. A QTc interval of 500 ms or greater is considered to be a high risk factor for torsades de pointes, though the prediction of arrhythmia is not simply linearly dependent on QT measure. An elevated risk of serious adverse cardiac events or sudden cardiac death has been documented for thioridazine, clozapine, droperidol, pimozide, and sertindole. These are considered higher-risk antipsychotics in terms of serious cardiac effects. Haloperidol, quetiapine, risperidone, chlorpromazine, and trifluoperazine have a tendency to extend the QT interval even at therapeutic doses, but their link with sudden cardiac death is not yet clarified. Amisulpride, aripiprazole, olanzapine, sulpride, and zotepine have not been linked with an elevated risk of sudden cardiac death or QTc prolongation. Typical neuroleptics that have lower potency, such as thioridazine and chlorpromazine, are more cardiotoxic than high-potency drugs such a haloperidol. The major effects on the electrocardiogram include prolongation of the QT and PR intervals, T wave blunting or inversion, and ST segment depression. Sudden death noted in antipsychotic recipients may also be due to seizures during sleep, sudden asphyxiation, temperature dysregulation (for example malignant hyperthermia), and neuroleptic malignant syndrome.

Abdelmawla N and Mitchell AJ. Sudden cardiac death and antipsychotics. Part 2: Monitoring and prevention. *Advances in Psychiatric Treatment* 2006; **12**: 100–109.

52. B. Drugs can undergo two different types of clearance when administered. When a constant fraction of a drug is cleared per unit time, it is called first-order kinetics. This means that when the amount of drug in plasma or dose of administered drug increases, the clearance proportionately increases as a stable fraction of plasma concentration. When the system facilitating such clearance of drugs becomes saturated, drugs follow zero-order kinetics. Here a constant amount, not a fraction, of the drug is cleared per unit time. This means that irrespective of the amount of drug in plasma or dose of drug administered, only a fixed unit of drug is cleared by the body. Thus, increasing the dose might result in serious toxicity in this case. Certain drugs have a propensity to undergo zero-order kinetics, even at therapeutic dose levels. Phenytoin metabolism is dose dependent, wherein smaller therapeutic doses follow first-order kinetics while higher doses follow zero-order kinetics. Gabapentin is not metabolized by liver and undergoes first-order renal clearance. Valproate follows first-order kinetics even in wide therapeutic dose levels. Lamotrigine, too, shows first-order linear kinetics and it is metabolized predominantly through glucuronidation.

Splinter MY. Pharmacokinetic properties of new antiepileptic drugs. *Journal of Pharmacy Practice* 2005; **18**: 444–460.

53. E. The small intestine has the largest surface area for drug absorption in the GI tract, and its membranes are more permeable than oral epithelium, oesophagus, or stomach. Hence most drugs are absorbed primarily in the small intestine. Gut mucosa harbours many metabolic enzymes that can breakdown active drug molecules and reduce the bioavailability of administered drugs.

Atkinson A *et al.*, eds. *Principles of Clinical Pharmacology*, 2nd edn. Elsevier, 2007, p. 39.

54. D. The abrupt discontinuance of SSRI use is associated with a discontinuation syndrome. This is characterized by fatigue, light headedness, nausea, headache, anxiety, insomnia and poor concentration, flu like symptoms, and electric shock-like paresthesias. In most cases, at least 6 weeks of treatment have elapsed before a discontinuation reaction takes place. The symptoms are self-resolving within 3 weeks in most cases. It is suggested that those who tolerate SSRIs poorly on initiation are more likely to develop discontinuation symptoms. Fluoxetine is the SSRI least likely to be associated with this syndrome, because it has a metabolite that is active with a half-life of more than a week. Shorter half-life medications, such as paroxetine, are associated with more discontinuation symptoms. Other classes of antidepressants, such as venlafaxine and tricyclics, are also associated with discontinuation reactions.

Taylor D *et al.*, eds. *The Maudsley Prescribing Guidelines*, 9th edn. Informa Healthcare, 2007, p. 240.

55. A. Paroxetine has a half-life of nearly 21 hours, which is short compared to fluoxetine, which has a prolonged duration of action due to an active metabolite that remains in the body for many days. In addition, paroxetine is more anticholinergic than most other SSRIs. Too rapid a discontinuation of any drug with significant anticholinergic properties may lead to a cholinergic rebound. The symptoms are characterized by acetylcholine excess—nausea, vomiting sweating, stomach cramps, diarrhoea, anxiety, agitation, and insomnia. In some cases delirium can result. This rebound is more common with tricyclics than SSRIs, except in the case of paroxetine which has significant anticholinergic effects.

Taylor D *et al.*, eds. *The Maudsley Prescribing Guidelines*, 9th edn. Informa Healthcare, 2007, p. 241.

56. A. Dosulepin or dothiepin together with amitriptyline has been associated with most cases of fatal tricyclic antidepressant overdose. The ingestion of large quantities of tricyclics in overdose results in complex changes in the normal pharmacokinetics observed at therapeutic doses. Due to anticholinergic effects, gastric emptying is delayed and a sustained slow absorption takes place. Respiratory depression produces acidosis, which reduces protein binding and increases the active free fraction of the toxic drug. The toxic effects of tricyclics are due mainly to an increased sympathetic drive, adrenergic blockade, arrythmogenic effect on myocardium, and anticholinergic action.

Kerr GW, McGuffie AC, and Wilkie S. Tricyclic antidepressant overdose: a review. *Emergency Medicine Journal* 2001; **18**: 236–241.

57. A. Many treatment variables are associated as risk factors for neuroleptic malignant syndrome (NMS). Nearly all dopamine antagonists have been associated with NMS, although high-potency conventional antipsychotics are associated with a greater risk compared with low-potency agents and atypical antipsychotics. Intramuscular administration, rapid tranquilization, and faster titration rates are associated with higher incidence. Drugs with an intrinsic anticholinergic property have a lower propensity to cause NMS. Atypical agents produce atypical NMS, where the classic rigidity or hyperthermia component of NMS may be conspicuously absent. The risk of NMS is not related to α adrenergic blockade or sedative property of an antipsychotic drug.

Stübner S, Rustenbeck E, Grohmann R *et al.* Severe and uncommon involuntary movement disorders due to psychotropic drugs. *Pharmacopsychiatry* 2004; **37** (Suppl. 1): S54–S64.

58. B. Benzodiazepine withdrawal symptoms include anxiety, inner tension, dizziness, insomnia, and anorexia. More severe withdrawal symptoms include nausea and vomiting, severe tremor, muscle weakness, postural hypotension, and tachycardia with psychological symptoms of dysphoria, depressive pessimistic thoughts, and obsessive ruminations. Myoclonus, pain symptoms, ataxia, kinaesthetic hallucinations, depersonalization, and hyperacusis are also noted. The withdrawal symptoms can develop after only 4 weeks of continuous use. Clonazepam, carbamazepine, and long-acting benzodiazepines themselves have been used in the management of withdrawal symptoms.

Taylor D et al., eds. *The Maudsley Prescribing Guidelines*, 9th edn. Informa Healthcare, 2007, p. 264.

59. B. Typical neuroleptics vary in their potential to cause anticholinergic symptoms. As a general rule, high-potency medications such as haloperidol produce less anticholinergic effects compared to low-potency drugs such as chlorpromazine and thioridazine. Peripheral anticholinergic effects include dry mouth, blurred vision, constipation, and urinary retention. Central anticholinergic effects, such as confusion and delirium, are seen especially in overdose of low-potency agents and in the elderly.

Sadock BJ and Sadock VA. *Kaplan and Sadock's Synopsis of Psychiatry: Behavioral Sciences/Clinical Psychiatry*, 10th edn. Lippincott Williams and Wilkins, 2007, p. 1048.

60. D. Severe sweating incongruent to room temperature is associated with TCAs, SSRIs, and venlafaxine. This is a socially disabling side-effect. Drugs such as terazosin, cyproheptadine, benztropine, and oxybutynin have been tried anecdotally to treat this symptom but none of these has been recommended for routine use. The mechanism by which SSRIs increase sweating is unknown but is hypothesized to be through activation of the sympathetic nervous system or by action on the hypothalamus.

Sadock BJ and Sadock VA. *Kaplan and Sadock's Synopsis of Psychiatry: Behavioral Sciences/Clinical Psychiatry*, 10th edn. Lippincott Williams and Wilkins, 2007, p. 983.
Marcy R and Britton ML. Antidepressant-induced sweating. *Annals of Pharmacotherapy* 2005; **39**: 748–752.

61. A. The most commonly used anticholinergic drugs for extrapyramidal symptoms in patients taking antipsychotics are trihexyphenidyl (benzhexol), benztropine, biperiden, and procyclidine. Orphenadrine is an antihistaminergic agent with prominent anticholinergic action. Benztropine also has some antihistaminergic effects. All these agents are antimuscarinic. Trihexyphenidyl (benzhexol) is the most stimulating of all anticholinergics.

Sadock BJ and Sadock VA. *Kaplan and Sadock's Synopsis of Psychiatry: Behavioral Sciences/Clinical Psychiatry*, 10th edn. Lippincott Williams and Wilkins, 2007, p. 1004.

62. C. Benztropine is the least stimulating anticholinergic agent and so it is least associated with drug-abuse potential. Benztropine reaches peak plasma concentrations in 2 to 3 hours after oral administration and acts for 1 to 12 hours. Benztropine is available as an intramuscular preparation and this is preferred when available in acute dystonia.

Sadock BJ and Sadock VA. *Kaplan and Sadock's Synopsis of Psychiatry: Behavioral Sciences/Clinical Psychiatry*, 10th edn. Lippincott Williams and Wilkins, 2007, p. 1004.

63. A. Trihexyphenidyl is suspected to have some dopaminergic activities which produce stimulating effects. It has a higher abuse potential than other anticholinergic drugs.

Smith JM. Abuse of the antiparkinson drugs: a review of the literature. *Journal of Clinical Psychiatry* 1980; **41**: 351–354.

64. E. Lithium-induced tremor is frequently postural in nature and occurs at 8 to 12 Hz frequency. It is most notable in outstretched hands. If troublesome, the tremor can be reduced by giving lithium in divided doses or using a sustained release formulation wherein peaks and troughs in plasma level are better managed. A reduction in tremors can be noted if the patient's anxiety is better managed and caffeine intake is reduced. β-blockers, such as propranolol, have been used to reduce lithium-induced tremor. If the tremors turn coarse, suspect lithium toxicity. Procyclidine can alleviate extrapyramidal symptoms but it has no effects on lithium-induced tremors.

Sadock BJ and Sadock VA. *Kaplan and Sadock's Synopsis of Psychiatry: Behavioral Sciences/Clinical Psychiatry*, 10th edn. Lippincott Williams and Wilkins, 2007, p. 1059.

65. A. Donepezil is an anticholinesterase drug widely used in patients with a moderate degree of Alzheimer's dementia. It is administered orally once daily. The half-life of donepezil is 70 hours in the elderly and steady-state levels are achieved within about 2 weeks. The half-life of rivastigmine, another antidementia drug, is 1 hour, but it dissociates slowly from cholinesterase enzyme, thus a single dose is therapeutically active for 10 hours. Rivastigmine is taken twice daily. Galantamine is an alkaloid (extracted from daffodils (*Narcissus pseudonarcissus*) and snow drops (*Galanthus nivalis*)); it has an elimination half-life of nearly 6 hours, and so is administered twice daily. A sustained release preparation is now available.

Sadock BJ and Sadock VA. *Kaplan and Sadock's Synopsis of Psychiatry: Behavioral Sciences/Clinical Psychiatry*, 10th edn. Lippincott Williams and Wilkins, 2007, p. 1034.

66. D. Alcohol (ethanol) is metabolized via an oxidation reaction catalysed by alcohol dehydrogenase. This results in formation of acetaldehyde, which is further broken down to acetyl-coenzyme A by aldehyde dehydrogenase. Disulfiram is a non-competitive, irreversible aldehyde dehydrogenase inhibitor. So when alcohol is taken together with disulfiram this leads to accumulation of acetaldehyde. A high level of acetaldehyde is associated with nausea, throbbing headache, vomiting, hypertension, flushing, sweating, thirst, dyspnoea, tachycardia, chest pain, vertigo, and blurred vision. The accumulation of acetaldehyde occurs almost immediately after the ingestion of alcohol in those who take disulfiram; the reaction can last from 30 minutes to 2 hours. The initiation of disulfiram should not take place unless the patient has abstained from alcohol for at least 12 hours. Its half-life is estimated to be 60 to 120 hours. The effect of disulfiram treatment can last as long as 1 or 2 weeks after the last dose of disulfiram. Most fatal reactions occur in persons who are taking more than 500 mg a day of disulfiram and who consume more than 90 g of alcohol.

Sadock BJ and Sadock VA. *Kaplan and Sadock's Synopsis of Psychiatry: Behavioral Sciences/Clinical Psychiatry*, 10th edn. Lippincott Williams and Wilkins, 2007, p. 1039.
Deitrich RA and Erwin VG. Mechanism of the inhibition of aldehyde dehydrogenase in vivo by disulfiram and diethyldithiocarbamate. *Molecular Pharmacology* 1971; **7**: 301–307.

67.A. Cigarette smoking occurs at a very high rate in patients with schizophrenia. Many reasons have been proposed as to why such high rates of smoking are seen in schizophrenia patients. One suggestion is that patients smoke as a form of self-medication with nicotine, which may help to regulate a dysfunctional mesolimbic dopamine system. Nicotine can increase dopamine release in the prefrontal cortex and reduce negative symptoms to some extent. Nicotine could enhance cognitive performance for certain tasks. Antipsychotic medications could block the dopamine reward pathway, necessitating an increase in nicotine concentrations needed to produce reward effects from smoking. Smoking may decrease the plasma levels of typical antipsychotic drugs via induction of the CYP450 enzymes system, providing some relief from extrapyramidal side-effects, but most patients who smoke start smoking even before onset of the illness.

Sadock BJ and Sadock VA. *Kaplan and Sadock's Synopsis of Psychiatry: Behavioral Sciences/Clinical Psychiatry*, 10th edn. Lippincott Williams and Wilkins, 2007, p. 1050.
Kelly C and McCreadie R. Cigarette smoking and schizophrenia. *Advances in Psychiatric Treatment* 2000; **6**: 327–331.

68. B. Acamprosate is a structural analogue of GABA and taurine. Its mechanism of action is thought to be antagonism of glutamatergic *N*-methyl-D-aspartate (NMDA) receptors. It should only be started after the individual has been successfully weaned off alcohol; this is not because of alcohol–acamprosate interaction but the efficacy of acamprosate is demonstrated only in individuals who have been successfully detoxified from alcohol. The concomitant intake of alcohol and acamprosate does not affect the pharmacokinetics of either alcohol or acamprosate, but if the patient relapses more than once while on acamprosate the treatment must be reconsidered. Administration of disulfiram does not affect the pharmacokinetics of acamprosate; though this is practiced at certain centres, no strong evidence exists to support the combination. Bupropion, used to aid abstinence from smoking, is started 2 weeks before a target date is set to quit smoking.

Sadock BJ and Sadock VA. *Kaplan and Sadock's Synopsis of Psychiatry: Behavioral Sciences/Clinical Psychiatry*, 10th edn. Lippincott Williams and Wilkins, 2007, p. 1039.

69. C. Dantrolene sodium is used to treat rigidity and hyperthermia in patients with neuroleptic malignant syndrome (NMS). Dantrolene binds to a calcium channel called ryanodine receptor in skeletal muscle, leading to a fall in intracellular calcium concentration and reduced contraction. It is usually administered via the intravenous route; it reduces muscle spasm in most patients with neuroleptic malignant syndrome. Dantrolene is not a stand-alone treatment for NMS; it must be accompanied by resuscitation, fluid replacement, and cardiac and respiratory support. Rigidity is relieved usually within minutes to hours of administration. Dantrolene can also be used in other cases of life-threatening muscle rigidity, for example catatonia and serotonin syndrome.

Sadock BJ and Sadock VA. *Kaplan and Sadock's Synopsis of Psychiatry: Behavioral Sciences/Clinical Psychiatry*, 10th edn. Lippincott Williams and Wilkins, 2007, p. 1037.

70. E. Haloperidol is chemically a butyrophenone. Fluphenazine, perphenazine, and trifluperazine are piperazine phenothiazines. Chlorpromazine is an aliphatic phenothiazine while thioridazine is a piperidine phenothiazine. Thiothixene is a thioxanthene antipsychotic; pimozide is a diphenyl butyl piperidine. Loxapine is a dibenzoxapine. Many of these typical antipsychotics are rarely used in current practice.

Sadock BJ and Sadock VA. *Kaplan and Sadock's Synopsis of Psychiatry: Behavioral Sciences/Clinical Psychiatry*, 10th edn. Lippincott Williams and Wilkins, 2007, p. 1047.

71. B. Lamotrigine is an anticonvulsant increasingly being used to prevent recurrent depressive episodes in bipolar disorder. Lamotrigine is thought to act via blockade of voltage-sensitive sodium channels, with secondary effect on calcium transport. Lamotrigine has weak effects on the serotonin system.

Sadock BJ and Sadock VA. *Kaplan and Sadock's Synopsis of Psychiatry: Behavioral Sciences/Clinical Psychiatry*, 10th edn. Lippincott Williams and Wilkins, 2007, p. 1054.

72. B. Lithium produces hypokalaemia-like changes on the electrocardiogram (ECG). This is related to displacement of intracellular potassium by the lithium ion. T-wave flattening or inversion is the commonest ECG change reported. These changes commonly disappear after stopping lithium. Lithium depresses the sinoatrial node; this can lead to sinus dysrhythmia, heart block, and syncope. Hence lithium is contraindicated in persons with sick sinus syndrome. Cardiac effects of lithium are more pronounced in those who have pre-existing cardiac problems, on diuretic treatment, and in those with renal impairment.

Sadock BJ and Sadock VA. *Kaplan and Sadock's Synopsis of Psychiatry: Behavioral Sciences/Clinical Psychiatry*, 10th edn. Lippincott Williams and Wilkins, 2007, p. 1059.

73. A. Lamotrigine is associated with rash, which is benign in about 8% of patients started on lamotrigine within the first 4 months of treatment. In a small but significant proportion of patients (nearly 0.1%) this may be an early manifestation of Stevens–Johnson syndrome or toxic epidermal necrolysis. So lamotrigine must be discontinued whenever a rash is reported during treatment. Unfortunately, this discontinuation is not always sufficient to prevent the life threatening-hypersensitivity reaction, Steven–Johnson syndrome. The chances of developing a rash increases if lamotrigine is started at a higher than recommended dose or titrated at a faster than recommended speed. Coadministration of valproate can also increase the incidence of rash.

Sadock BJ and Sadock VA. *Kaplan and Sadock's Synopsis of Psychiatry: Behavioral Sciences/Clinical Psychiatry*, 10th edn. Lippincott Williams and Wilkins, 2007, p. 1054.

74. A. The electrical stimulus delivered via ECT must be strong enough to reach the seizure threshold of the patient. Each individual has a different seizure threshold with nearly 40-fold variability among patients. During the course of ECT treatment itself, the seizure threshold could increase in the range of 25 to 200%. Older men generally have a higher threshold than the young. Amnesia related to ECT is proportional to the degree to which the administered electricity dose is high in relation to patients' seizure thresholds. Incidence of cognitive disturbance is higher when a patient receives thrice-weekly ECT compared to twice-weekly treatments.

UK ECT Review Group. Efficacy and safety of electroconvulsive therapy in depressive disorders: a systematic review and meta-analysis. *Lancet* 2003; **361**: 799–808.

75. B. Bupropion resembles amphetamine in its structure—it is a monocyclic aminoketone. Bupropion is a norepinephrine and dopamine reuptake inhibitor. Its side-effects profile is different from that of SSRIs in that it causes very low incidence of sexual dysfunction or sedation and produces some weight loss. It does not cause significant discontinuation reactions. It is currently licensed to help people quit smoking, but is not licensed as an antidepressant in the UK. Bupropion is contraindicated in patients with a history of eating disorder; it can cause significant changes in appetite. Bupropion has a high propensity to cause seizures.

Sadock BJ and Sadock VA. *Kaplan and Sadock's Synopsis of Psychiatry: Behavioral Sciences/Clinical Psychiatry*, 10th edn. Lippincott Williams and Wilkins, 2007, p. 1024.

76. D. In the UK, duloxetine is marketed to treat stress urinary incontinence (SUI) in women under the name Yentreve® (Eli Lilly and Company). The female urethra has a rhabdosphincter of circularly arranged striated muscles. Generally, relaxation of this sphincter allows micturition. The sphincter is innervated by neurones from the sacral spinal cord (S2–S4). Duloxetine blocks the reuptake of serotonin and norepinephrine at this site to stimulate contraction of the rhabdosphincter, leading to an increase in the tone of the urethral sphincter. The increased muscle tone inhibits involuntary urine loss. To treat stress incontinence, a dose of 40 mg twice daily (80 mg/day) is recommended. In depression a dose of 60 mg/day given once daily is often used. Duloxetine can also help neuropathic pain, where a higher dose of up to 120 mg has been used.

Thor KB. Serotonin and norepinephrine involvement in efferent pathways to the urethral rhabdosphincter: implications for treating stress urinary incontinence. *Urology* 2003; **62**: 3–9.

77. C. Lamotrigine is mainly metabolized via glucuronidation and does not have much effect on other prescribed medications, but valproate has been observed to double the plasma levels of lamotrigine. The elimination half-life of lamotrigine in healthy young adults is approximately 25 to 30 hours. In patients taking valproate this is prolonged to 60 hours. As a result, when lamotrigine is initiated for patients who are taking valproate, the starting dose should be approximately 50% of the normal starting dose of lamotrigine. Some suggest that if valproate is started for a patient who is already on lamotrigine, one must consider obtaining a baseline lamotrigine plasma concentration. The lamotrigine dose may have to be reduced during the valproate dose titration. As a result of this interaction, the incidence of lamotrigine-induced rash seems to be more common in those taking the combination. Phenytoin, carbamazepine, and oral contraceptives may reduce the half-life of lamotrigine.

Anderson GD, Yau MK, Gidal BE *et al.* Bidirectional interaction of valproate and lamotrigine in healthy subjects. *Clinical Pharmacology and Theraputics* 1996; **60**: 145–156.

78. A. Lithium can aggravate psoriasis. The induction of psoriasis without pre-existing disease is less common than exacerbation of existing disease. Not all patients with pre-existing psoriasis have a flare when starting lithium and psoriasis is not considered to be a contraindication to taking lithium for mania or depression. Similarly, other drugs such as β-blockers, antimalarials, and indometacin can aggravate psoriasis. Psoriasis that has flared with lithium appears to be more resistant to standard treatment modalities. Some preliminary evidence suggests that supplemental inositol or omega-3-fatty acids may improve symptoms in patients with psoriasis during lithium treatment. Histological studies on the skin lesions induced or aggravated by lithium are equivocal; some support the lesions to be consistent with psoriasis, although others have claimed the features as non-specific and refer to as psoriasiform dermatitis.

Fry L and Baker BS. Triggering psoriasis: the role of infections and medications. *Clinics in Dermatology* 2007; **25**: 606–615.

79. C. Ployuria, one of the most common side-effects of lithium, is related to tubular concentrating defect that is resistant to vasopressin. This results in nephrogenic diabetes insipidus. Vasopressin receptor expression is reduced by lithium, leading to a failure of facilitation of water movement. It is thought that taking lithium in a single dose prevents, or at least limits, renal tubular impairment. The most likely reason for the reduction of thirst and polyuria is the less frequent stimulation of the thirst centre by the lithium salts in once-a-day doses. However, some studies have shown that the beneficial effect of single dosage is seen only in those who received multiple doses for a short time. It is possible that long-term, multiple-dose administration results in irreversible changes in tubular mechanisms. Patient adherence can be improved by a single-dosing schedule of lithium; however, once-a-day schedules have not been shown to be conclusively superior with respect to glomerular damage or renal failure.

Ljubicic D, Letica-Crepulja M, Vitezic D et al. Lithium treatments: single and multiple daily dosing. *Canadian Journal of Psychiatry* 2008; **53**: 323–331.

80. E. On pharmacokinetic grounds, oxazepam may be preferable to chlordiazepoxide in cirrhotic patients since the elimination of oxazepam is not greatly altered in cirrhosis. In general, longer-acting benzodiazepines, such as chlordiazepoxide or diazepam, are preferred as they produce a smoother withdrawal course with less breakthrough or rebound symptoms, but they may lead to excess sedation for patients with hepatic dysfunction/cirrhosis. Shorter-acting benzodiazepines, such as oxazepam, may result in greater discomfort and more discharges against medical advice, because alcohol withdrawal symptoms tend to recur when the plasma drug levels drop. Shorter-acting agents, such as lorazepam or oxazepam, require more frequent dosing. They may be more useful for symptom-triggered regimens than fixed-dose regimens of alcohol detoxification.

Taylor D et al., eds. *The Maudsley Prescribing Guidelines*, 9th edn. Informa Healthcare, 2007, p. 237.

81. D. Anticholinergic drugs may exacerbate some symptoms of tardive dyskinesia (TD). Traditionally, long-term anticholinergic prescriptions are thought to promote the onset of TD, though the evidence in support of this notion is minimal. Tardive dyskinesia is a troublesome side-effect of antipsychotics. It is more common in older patients and those with neurological diseases. The risk of tardive dyskinesia is estimated as 3–5% per year of exposure (at least for the first 5 years) with conventional antipsychotics. The appearance of symptoms usually takes more than 3 months, the risk increasing proportionally with duration of treatment. In elderly patients this increases to be as high as 25% within the first year of exposure to typical antipsychotics. Women, children, and patients with primary mood disorders or learning disabilities are also at higher risk. Some studies report an increased risk associated with diabetes and comorbid substance use.

Tasman A, Maj M et al., eds. *Psychiatry*, 3rd edn. John Wiley and Sons, 2008, p. 1783.

82. B. Serotonin is released from platelets in response to vascular injury. It promotes vasoconstriction and platelet aggregation. Platelets do not possess the synthetic machinery to produce serotonin and so depend on uptake via 5-HT transporters on their membrane. SSRIs inhibit the serotonin transporter, leading to a hyposerotonergic state in platelets. This reduces the ability to form clots, with subsequent increase in the risk of bleeding. Thus, SSRIs cause a functional impairment of platelet aggregation (thrombasthenia), but not a reduction in platelet number. This can cause easy bruising or prolonged bleeding in those with gastric ulcers or bleeding diathesis. Some authors recommend gastroprotection when SSRIs are coadministered with NSAIDs.

Paton C and Ferrier IN. SSRIs and gastrointestinal bleeding. *BMJ* 2005; **331**: 529–530.

83. A.   Varenicline is a partial agonist at the $\alpha_4\beta_2$ unit of the nicotinic acetylcholine receptor. It is shown to assist smoking cessation by relieving nicotine withdrawal symptoms and reducing the rewarding properties of nicotine. It is advised to choose a quitting date and start taking the tablets 1 week before the date. Generally, varenicline is started at 0.5 mg daily, increasing to 0.5 mg twice daily after 3 days. The final dose is 1 mg twice daily for up to 12 weeks.

Jorenby DE, Hays JT, Rigotti NA *et al.* Efficacy of varenicline, an $\alpha_4\beta_2$ nicotinic acetylcholine receptor partial agonist, vs placebo or sustained-release bupropion for smoking cessation: a randomized controlled trial. *JAMA* 2006; **296**: 56–63.

84. E.   All of the listed drugs except α_1-blockers are associated with erectile dysfunction. Parasympathetic activity during arousal triggers the release of nitric oxide, which increases the levels of the intracellular cyclic guanosine monophosphate (cGMP). Increases in cGMP cause penile vascular and trabecular smooth muscle relaxation, leading to increase in blood flow. The rapid filling of the cavernosal spaces compresses venules leading to reduction in venous outflow. This process effectively raises intracavernosal pressure, resulting in erection. α_1 adrenergic blockers can enhance erectile function by reducing the sympathetic tone and relaxing trabecular smooth muscle cells. Nearly 25% of cases of erectile dysfunction are related to medication side-effects. Many prescribed drugs, including β-blockers, H_2 antagonists, diuretics, antiepileptics, antidepressants, and antiparkinsonian medications, can cause erectile dysfunction. In addition, street drugs such as cannabis, cocaine, alcohol, ecstasy, and opiates can also lead to impotence.

Tasman A, Maj M *et al.*, eds. *Psychiatry*, 3rd edn. John Wiley and Sons, 2008, p. 1588.

85. B.   The vasodilatation required to bring on erection is mediated by nitric oxide (NO). Nitric oxide enables vascular smooth muscle relaxation via production of a second messenger, called cGMP. Men suffering from erectile dysfunction (ED) may have successful erection if the availability of cGMP is prolonged or increased. This can be achieved by modulating an enzyme called phosphodiesterase (PDE-5). Normally PDE-5 terminates the action of cGMP by converting it into inactive form (GMP). By inhibiting PDE-5, sildenafil lengthens the life of cGMP and helps to achieve erection.

There are nine different types of PDE found in different tissues of the body; for example coronary tissues have the PDE-3 type receptors; PDE-5 receptors are found in platelets and various muscle tissues; and PDE-6 receptors are found in the retina. Sildenafil has some propensity to act on PDE-6, apart from its primary action on PDE-5; this explains defects in colour vision experienced by some patients taking sildenafil. As sildenafil does not produce new cGMP directly, it cannot act as an aphrodisiac. Hence it cannot help patients with reduced arousal due to other causes such as depression.

Francis SH and Corbin JD. Sildenafil: efficacy, safety, tolerability and mechanism of action in treating erectile dysfunction. *Expert Opinion on Drug Metabolism and Toxicology* 2005; **1**: 283–293.

86. D. Naloxone is an opioid antagonist and has no analgesic activities. Naltrexone is a longer-acting opioid antagonist with no clinically useful analgesic actions. Nomifensine is not an opioid; it is a cyclic antidepressant with norepinephrine and dopamine reuptake inhibition. It was withdrawn from the clinical market due to hepatotoxicity and renal damage, in addition to fears regarding abuse potential. Propoxyphene has mild to moderate analgesic properties but its metabolite, norpropoxyphene, is devoid of clinically useful analgesia. Codeine, on the other hand, is a strong analgesic and breaks down to morphine which has potent analgesic activity. Codeine is ineffective as an analgesic at usual doses in 7 to 10% of the white population with low activity *CYP2D6* alleles. It is reported that in those with ultrarapid CYP2D6 metabolism, codeine intake may result in an increase in morphine production, occasionally resulting in opioid intoxication.

Yue QY, Alm C, Svensson JO, and Sawe J. Quantification of the O- and N-demethylated and the glucuronidated metabolites of codeine relative to the debrisoquine metabolic ratio in urine in ultrarapid, rapid, and poor debrisoquine hydroxylators. *Therapeutic Drug Monitoring* 1997; **19**: 539–542.

87. C. There are three important types of opioid receptors; most analgesic effects are associated with μ receptors. The δ and κ receptors also contribute to the analgesic effect to some extent. Morphine and codeine mainly act via μ receptors to produce clinical analgesia. Opioids are coupled to Gi proteins that decrease cAMP. When opioids bind to μ receptors, hyperpolarization of the nociceptive neurone (sensory neurone for pain) takes place via opening of K^+ channels and inhibition of the Ca^{2+} channels. This reduces neuronal activity and reduces the transmission of pain signals via ascending pathways to the brain.

Stein C, Schäfer M, and Machelska H. Attacking pain at its source: new perspectives on opioids. *Nature Medicine* 2003; **9**: 1003–1008.

88. B. Methylxanthines include caffeine and theophylline. They have CNS stimulatory properties. At therapeutic doses, these drugs block adenosine receptors; at higher concentrations inhibition of the phosphodiesterase enzyme takes place. Adenosine is released from neurones and glia. It acts via G-protein-coupled receptors (A_1, A_{2A}, A_{2B}, and A_3). A_1 receptors have inhibitory role while A_2 receptors have stimulatory properties. A_1 receptor antagonism may enhance cognition and facilitate arousal. At higher doses where inhibition of phosphodiesterase occurs, intracellular levels of cAMP increase.

Abbracchio MP and Cattabeni F. Brain adenosine receptors as targets for therapeutic intervention in neurodegenerative diseases. *Annals of the New York Academy of Science* 1999; **890**: 79–92.

89. C. Livedo reticularis refers to a characteristic purple mottling of the skin see in patients taking amantadine. It is usually seen as a lacy, net-like pattern of vascular change on the legs. It is also associated with vasculitis such as lupus. Mostly, the livedo reticularis disappears when the drug is discontinued, usually within several weeks. The appearance of livedo does not always warrant the cessation of the drug. The common side-effects of levodopa include insomnia, postural hypotension, gastrointestinal disturbances, tremors, mood changes, and fatigue. Bromocriptine can cause postural hypotension, nausea, oedema, confusion, dry mouth, and depression. Tolcapone is a COMT inhibitor and can cause abdominal pain, back pain, constipation, nausea, diarrhoea, and liver failure.

Sladden MJ, Nicolaou N, Johnston GA *et al*. Livedo reticularis induced by amantadine. *British Journal of Dermatology* 2003; **149**: 656–658.

90. D. Tiagabine is an add-on antiepileptic drug developed by modifying a GABA uptake inhibitor called nipecotic acid. Tiagabine is a potent inhibitor of GABA uptake into both neurones and glial cells. It acts via selective inhibition of the GABA transporter, GAT-1. Through this mechanism, tiagabine enhances $GABA_A$ receptor-mediated tonic inhibition. Vigabatrin is a selective and irreversible GABA-transaminase inhibitor. Topiramate produces its antiepileptic effect through several mechanisms such as modification of Na^+-dependent and/or Ca^{2+}-dependent action potentials, enhancement of GABA-mediated Cl^- fluxes into neurones, and inhibition of kainate-mediated conductance at AMPA glutamate receptors. Gabapentin is a structural analogue of GABA and though originally designed as a GABA-mimetic, its mechanism of action is still unknown.

Perucca E. Clinical pharmacology and therapeutic use of the new antiepileptic drugs. *Fundamental and Clinical Pharmacology* 2001; **15**: 405–417.

91. A. Melatonin has not been demonstrated to have clinically significant antidepressant properties. Ropinirole is a dopamine agonist; it acts via the stimulation of postsynaptic dopamine D_2-type receptors within the basal ganglia. Agomelatine is a novel agent promoted as a melatonergic antidepressant; its main antidepressant effect is mediated via $5-HT_{2C}$ antagonism, which may modulate noradrenergic and dopaminergic neurotransmission. L-tryptophan is a serotonin precursor and is not considered as melatonergic drug. Modafinil is not used as an antidepressant; it acts via an influence on dopamine-dependent adrenergic signalling, though the exact mechanism is still unclear.

Palaniyappan L and McAllister-Williams RH. Antidepressants: will new mechanisms of action improve poor outcomes? *British Journal of Hospital Medicine* (Lond) 2008; **69**: 88–90.

92. D. Buprenorphine and naloxone act via opioid receptors; they are not indicated in sleep disorders such as narcolepsy. Antidepressants, including fluoxetine and tricyclics such as imipramine, can help cataplexy (sudden loss of muscle tone) in narcolepsy. Modafinil is a drug with stimulant properties and it is used to promote wakefulness in narcolepsy and allied disorders.

Dauvilliers Y, Arnulf I, and Mignot E. Narcolepsy with cataplexy. *Lancet* 2007; **369**: 499–511.

93. D. Pindolol acts as a partial agonist at $5-HT_{1A}$ receptors. Several controlled studies in the past have shown that the addition of pindolol to SSRI therapy rapidly potentiates the effects of these antidepressants. However, despite the rapidity of improvement with the combination, most studies found no overall advantage at the end of the study period. Systematic review of randomized controlled trials does not support the use of pindolol and β-blockers are not licensed for the treatment of depression. Pentazocine is a partial agonist at kappa opiate receptors; it has some psychotomimetic properties but is not used as an antidepressant. In fact, it may induce depression. Tramadol is an opioid analgesic with no antidepressant effects.

Stimpson N, Agrawal N, and Lewis G. Randomized controlled trials investigating pharmacological and psychological interventions for treatment-refractory depression. Systematic review. *British Journal of Psychiatry* 2002; **181**: 284–294.

94. E.   The mean elimination half-life of atomoxetine after oral administration is 5.2 hours. In poor metabolizers (CYP2D6 polymorphism) the mean elimination half-life is more than 20 hours, due to reduced clearance. Nearly 80% of atomoxetine is excreted in the urine. Atomoxetine does not affect the cytochrome P450 2D6 enzyme system. The effects of atomoxetine last longer than would be expected from its half-life; hence, once-daily administration is effective.

Barton, J. Atomoxetine: a new pharmacotherapeutic approach in the management of attention deficit/hyperactivity disorder. *Archives of Diseases in Childhood* 2005; **90** (Suppl. I): i26–i29.

95. C.   Antidepressant combinations involving MAOIs require close monitoring due to the risk of serotonergic and hypertensive side-effects. Phenelzine is supposed to be the safest MAO-A inhibitor in combination therapy for depression. It is a derivative of hydrazine similar to isonaizid, but the latter is mainly used as an antituberculosis drug and has only a weak antidepressant action. Selegeline is an MAO-B inhibitor.

Palaniyappan L, Insole L, and Ferrier IN. Combining antidepressants: a review of evidence. *Advances in Psychiatric Treatment* 2009; **15**: 90–99.

1. A 64-year-old lady, on physical examination exhibits symptoms suggestive of a movement disorder with associated speech deficits. This clinical presentation is classified as 'hypokinetic dysarthria' by her neurologist. It is associated with
   A. Parkinson's disease
   B. Huntington's disease
   C. Spasmodic dysphonia
   D. Multiple sclerosis
   E. Myasthenia gravis

2. A 32-year-old man is diagnosed with a right-sided hemiparesis. On examination, his speech shows non-fluent aphasia. His comprehension is intact, but repetition is impaired. He is most likely to have
   A. Transcortical motor aphasia
   B. Transcortical sensory aphasia
   C. Conduction aphasia
   D. Broca's aphasia
   E. Wernicke's aphasia

3. A patient presents with features suggestive of Gerstmann's syndrome. He also has aphasia. Which of the following is the most likely type of aphasia with which he may present?
   A. Transcortical sensory aphasia
   B. Transcortical motor aphasia
   C. Anomic aphasia
   D. Global aphasia
   E. Broca's aphasia

4. Regarding aphasia, which of the following statements is true?
   A. Broca's aphasia presents with logorrhoea.
   B. Neologism is a feature of Broca's aphasia.
   C. Paragrammatism is a feature of Wernicke's aphasia.
   D. Pure word deafness is associated with loss of naming.
   E. Involvement of the posterior cerebral artery leads to global aphasia.

5. **Which of the following is true regarding acquired defects in reading and writing?**
    A. Alexia without agraphia is called acquired illiteracy.
    B. Alexia without agraphia is seen in association with Gerstmann's syndrome.
    C. Anomic aphasia is associated with Gerstmann's syndrome.
    D. Transcortical aphasia is due to lesions in the arcuate fasciculus.
    E. Alexia without agraphia is seen in posterior cerebral artery stroke.

6. **The clinical sign of finger–nose ataxia is seen in lesions of which of the following structures?**
    A. Superior colliculus
    B. Inferior colliculus
    C. Pyramidal decussation
    D. Inferior olivary nucleus
    E. Thalamus

7. **A patient is observed to be repeating the phrases or words spoken by the examiner. Which of the following can cause this phenomenon?**
    A. Transcortical motor aphasia
    B. Transcortical sensory aphasia
    C. Mixed transcortical aphasia
    D. Huntington's disease
    E. All of the above

8. **Neuropsychiatric Interview (NPI) is often employed in patients with dementia or cognitive deterioration to detect psychiatric and behavioural problems. Which of the following is not tested by the NPI?**
    A. Thought disturbance
    B. Perceptual disturbance
    C. Affective disturbance
    D. Abnormalities in sleep pattern
    E. Disorientation

9. **Regarding handedness, which of these statements is true?**
    A. The population can be divided into two categories: right and left handed.
    B. 60% of the population are right handed.
    C. 75% of right-handed people are left-hemisphere dominant for language.
    D. 60% of left-handed people are left-hemisphere dominant for language.
    E. Left-handed people are less likely than right-handed ones to have bilateral language representation.

10. **A patient with a history of traumatic brain injury undergoes neuropsychological testing. In part A of the test he is asked to connect numbered circles on a paper as fast as he can in correct order, using a pen. In part B of the same test the same task is repeated but numbers and alphabets occur in alternate sequences. Which of the following statements is correct with regard to this test?**

A. This is called letter cancellation task.
B. This test is not sensitive to progressive cognitive decline in dementia.
C. Part A of the test corresponds more closely to executive functioning than part B.
D. Patients with traumatic injury perform this test slower than average.
E. This is purely a test of selective attention.

11. **Which of the following matches is incorrect regarding amnestic syndrome and site of lesion?**

A. Wernicke–Korsakoff syndrome–thalamic nuclei
B. Herpes simplex encephalitis–anterior temporal cortex
C. Crutzfeld–Jakob disease–diffuse cortical
D. Anterior communicating artery stroke–medial temporal cortex
E. Complex partial seizures–hippocampal damage

12. **Which of the following is a component of the triad in Balint's syndrome?**

A. Visual neglect
B. Achromatopsia
C. Prosopagnosia
D. Simultanagnosia
E. Anosognosia

13. **Features of Gerstmann's syndrome include all of the following except**

A. Dysgraphia
B. Finger agnosia
C. Dysarthria
D. Inability to distinguish left from right
E. Acalculia

14. **Blindsight is a feature of which of the following focal cortical syndromes?**

A. Balint's syndrome
B. Geschwind's syndrome
C. Charcot–Willibrand syndrome
D. Anton's syndrome
E. Central achromatopsia

15. **A patient is not able to perform sequential motor acts despite intact comprehension, muscle power, and ability to perform single-step commands. He is exhibiting**

    A. Ideational apraxia
    B. Ideomotor apraxia
    C. Conceptual apraxia
    D. Conduction apraxia
    E. Dissociation apraxia

16. **Which of the following is true about limb-kinetic apraxia?**

    A. Tasks such as finger tapping and pegboard are typically unimpaired.
    B. Picking up objects using pincer grasp is spared.
    C. It usually affects the hand that is ipsilateral to a hemispheric lesion.
    D. The lesion is localized to the contralateral premotor cortex.
    E. Patients typically present with an inability to perform multistep motor task.

17. **Which of the following refers to defective recognition of sensory stimuli despite having intact sensory pathways?**

    A. Agnosia
    B. Alexia
    C. Anosognosia
    D. Apraxia
    E. Abulia

18. **A 55-year-old man finds it difficult to recognize faces. On further testing, his ability to discriminate faces and match faces is intact. The most likely condition he is suffering from is**

    A. Apperceptive prosopagnosia
    B. Associative prosopagnosia
    C. Apperceptive visual object agnosia
    D. Simultanagnosia
    E. Central achromatopsia

19. **Which of the following is true regarding episodic memory?**

    A. Episodic memory is implicit and non-declarative.
    B. Episodic memory loss is not seen without medial temporal lesions.
    C. Episodic memory loss can present as anterograde or retrograde amnesia.
    D. Episodic memory applies only to events of personal significance.
    E. Episodic memory is more often preserved than semantic memory in dementia.

20. During bedside cognitive testing, a 40-year-old patient is asked to give the years when World War II took place. Which of the following memories is tested here?
    A. Procedural memory
    B. Episodic memory
    C. Semantic memory
    D. Implicit memory
    E. Non-declarative memory

21. A 35-year-old woman recently separated from her boyfriend of 5 years was brought to the A&E with loss of memory. On examination, her memory loss is specific to events associated with her boy friend. But she remembers other events that took place around the same time. She is most probably suffering from
    A. Localized amnesia
    B. Selective amnesia
    C. Generalized amnesia
    D. Continuous amnesia
    E. Systematized amnesia

22. After an enjoyable evening with friends at a pub, Tom calculates the cost of the number of drinks that he had, subtracts the total from the value of money he gave the bartender, and calculates the change that is due. The system of memory that enables such calculation is
    A. Episodic memory
    B. Semantic memory
    C. Procedural memory
    D. Working memory
    E. Retrograde memory

23. Which of the following conditions does not show predominant abnormality in procedural memory?
    A. Parkinson's disease
    B. Huntington's disease
    C. Progressive supranuclear palsy
    D. Olivopontocerebellar degeneration
    E. Early Alzheimer's disease

24. **A patient who had developed a pyloric stenosis following ingestion of sulphuric acid develops a confusional state, ophthalmoplegia, and ataxia. Which of the following is not true?**

    A. A CT scan may reveal bilateral hypodense areas in the medial thalamus.
    B. The patient may present with difficulty in learning new information.
    C. Administration of thiamine in the acute phase may prevent the emergence of chronic amnesic syndrome.
    D. Confabulation is most common in the early stage of the amnesic syndrome.
    E. The patient's memory of events before the onset of amnesia is always normal.

25. **Which of the following is the least valuable clinical indicator of severity of head injury?**

    A. Duration of retrograde amnesia
    B. Glasgow Coma Scale
    C. Duration of unconsciousness
    D. Neurological lesions noted using an MRI
    E. Duration of post-traumatic amnesia

26. **A 24-year-old patient is admitted to a head injury unit following a road traffic accident. He recovers well from acute neurological deficits but is diagnosed with post-concussion syndrome. Which of the following statements pertaining to his condition is true?**

    A. There is a consistent relationship between severity of injury and the presence of post-concussion syndrome.
    B. Diplopia is an early symptom of post-concussion syndrome.
    C. CT scans show brain lesions in up to 50% of patients in the first week.
    D. Psychological factors are more likely to play a role in illnesses of shorter duration.
    E. There is no association between the presence of symptoms and compensatory claims.

27. **A 30-year-old man who was involved in a road traffic accident was unconscious for 10 minutes. His CT scan was normal and he is now conscious, but complaining of a bad headache. The family is concerned about him developing seizures as his father has a history of epilepsy. What is the next line of action?**

    A. Start phenytoin for 1 to 2 weeks
    B. Start prophylactic carbamazepine for a year
    C. Start long-term benzodiazepines
    D. An abnormal EEG in this patient is an indication for starting prophylactic antiepileptic medication
    E. Antiepileptics are not indicated

28. **A 25-year-old patient presented with a history of recurrent, unilateral visual disturbances that resolved completely, on-and-off episodes of pins and needles in her left hand, and recent-onset bladder disturbances. Which of the following statements regarding this illness is true?**

    A. The risk of her developing a major depressive disorder is 5–10% during her lifetime.
    B. Her likelihood of developing suicidal ideation is similar to that in the general population.
    C. She is 10 times more likely to develop a manic episode compared to the general population.
    D. Pathological laughing and crying is seen in around 10% of cases.
    E. There is no risk of triggering a relapse of neurological condition with ECT.

29. **Which of the following statements regarding cognitive impairment in multiple sclerosis is true?**

    A. Cognitive deficits are secondary to depressive symptoms.
    B. Cognitive deficits are closely related to physical disability and duration of illness.
    C. Memory deficits in multiple sclerosis are more apparent on recall compared to recognition.
    D. MMSE is a good test to screen for cognitive deficits in multiple sclerosis.
    E. Donepezil has not been found to be useful in improving memory in multiple sclerosis.

30. **Which of the following statements regarding pathological laughing and crying is true?**

    A. It is always associated with motor deficits such as pseudobulbar palsy.
    B. Exaggerated crying and laughing is attributed to an underlying mood disorder.
    C. Antidepressants have been found to be of no use in treatment.
    D. It has been associated with frontal executive function deficits.
    E. By definition, patients cannot have a comorbid mood disorder.

31. **Consciousness is preserved in which of the following types of seizures?**

    A. Tonic–clonic seizures
    B. Simple partial seizures
    C. Status epilepticus
    D. Absence seizures
    E. Complex partial seizures

32. **A 45-year-old lady developed recurrent seizures with aura, automatism, and lip smacking. Ictal EEG showed spike and sharp waves complex along the right temporal region. Which of the following statements regarding her diagnosis is not true?**

    A. The aura itself constitute a simple partial seizure.
    B. This presentation is highly suggestive of complex partial seizure.
    C. There is an increased chance of this lady developing mania in her lifetime.
    D. A right-sided focus increases the risk of depression compared to mania.
    E. There is a five-times increase in the risk of suicide compared to the general population.

33. **Features suggestive of Geschwind's syndrome include all except**
    A. Circumstantiality
    B. Hypographia
    C. Hyper-religiosity
    D. Viscosity
    E. Increased aggression

34. **A 23-year-old patient previously diagnosed with epilepsy presents to casualty with intractable seizures following the breakup of a relationship. She has been compliant on her medications. The neurologist suspects psychogenic non-epileptic seizures. Which of the following statements is true with regard to her condition?**
    A. A postictal prolactin elevation of two times the baseline level is reliable in diagnosing true seizures.
    B. Up to 80% of patients with seizures have psychogenic non-epileptic seizures.
    C. Less than 5% of cases with intractable seizures have psychogenic non-epileptic seizures.
    D. Presence of tongue bite and incontinence is diagnostic of true seizures.
    E. Video EEG recording is the gold standard for diagnosing psychogenic non-epileptic seizures.

35. **Early onset of major depression is most commonly associated with stroke pertaining to which of the following regions of the brain?**
    A. Right anterior
    B. Right posterior
    C. Left anterior
    D. Left posterior
    E. Bilateral posterior

36. **A 67-year-old business man is admitted to a stroke unit. He is having significant aphasia. He has episodes of anger outburst when someone tries to communicate with him. Which of the following is false regarding this 'catastrophic reaction'?**
    A. Family history of psychiatric disorders is more common in those with catastrophic reaction.
    B. It is associated with the presence of major depression.
    C. The reaction is mostly secondary to the presence of aphasia.
    D. Patients are more likely to have a personal history of psychiatric disorders.
    E. Higher frequency of basal ganglia lesions may be seen.

37. **Which of the following statements about poststroke depression is true?**
    A. Younger age predisposes to poststroke depression.
    B. Cortical atrophy prior to stroke predisposes to poststroke depression.
    C. Male sex is a risk factor for poststroke depression.
    D. Lower educational status is a risk factor for poststroke depression.
    E. Lower socioeconomic status is a risk factor for poststroke depression.

38. **A 67-year-old patient with stroke has left inferior quadrantanopia, left hemineglect, and dressing apraxia with mild hemiparesis on neurological examination. Which artery is most likely to be involved in the stroke?**

   A. Posterior cerebral artery
   B. Middle cerebral artery
   C. Anterior cerebral artery
   D. Common carotid artery
   E. Internal carotid artery

39. **Which of the following stages of sleep is characterized by more than 50% delta activity in the EEG?**

   A. Stage 1 NREM
   B. Stage 2 NREM
   C. Stage 3 NREM
   D. Stage 4 NREM
   E. REM sleep

40. **All the following are features of REM sleep except**

   A. Low brain oxygen consumption
   B. High cerebral blood flow
   C. Penile erection
   D. Absent electrodermal activity
   E. Dream-like mental state

41. **Regarding sleep terror, which of the following statements is false?**

   A. It is associated with REM sleep disturbance.
   B. Vocalizations may occur during the episode.
   C. There is usually amnesia for these episodes.
   D. It becomes exacerbated by sleep deprivation.
   E. It is associated with psychopathology in adults.

42. **A 25-year-old man complains of excessive daytime sleepiness. He loses balance and falls down every time he laughs at a joke. He also complains of seeing 'ghosts' while falling asleep. Which of the following is likely to be found in this patient?**

   A. A sleep-onset slow wave stage
   B. Excess of hypocretin in the hypothalamus
   C. Seizure activity on electroencephalography
   D. Episodes of sleep paralysis
   E. Absence of REM on polysomnography

43. **All of the following increases the risk of developing dementia in those with Parkinson's disease except**

    A. Older age group
    B. Greater severity of motor disturbances
    C. Longer duration of Parkinson's disease
    D. Being female
    E. Significant functional disability

44. **Which of the following is considered as a 'Parkinson plus' syndrome?**

    A. Wilson's disease
    B. Fredreich's ataxia
    C. Progressive supranuclear palsy
    D. Amyotrophic lateral sclerosis
    E. Guillain–Barré syndrome

45. **A 64-year-old man presents with sudden-onset blindness that started as a 'curtain coming down' and he lost his vision completely for a few minutes. Within 15 minutes this improved and was restored to full, normal vision. The origin of emboli in this case is most likely to be at**

    A. Posterior cerebral artery
    B. Anterior cerebral artery
    C. Internal carotid artery
    D. Anterior communicating artery
    E. Middle cerebral artery

46. **A 21-year-old lady is found wandering at a public place. She is unaware of her address or any other personal details. She was admitted and later found to be on the missing persons register at a police station 100 miles away. After 4 weeks, she regains normal memory and remembers having lost her mother in a fire accident 6 weeks ago. Which of the following is true about the nature of her memory problems?**

    A. Total amnesia for past events may be seen during the episode.
    B. No amnesia for the episode will be present following recovery.
    C. A vascular aetiology is most likely.
    D. Inability to learn new materials will be seen during the episode.
    E. Episodes are often accompanied by other neurological symptoms.

47. **A 63-year-old man with alcohol dependence suffers a serious head injury. On recovery he is found to have unusual behaviours. When a tooth brush is placed in front of him, he immediately begins to brush his teeth, even in entirely inappropriate contexts. He is exhibiting**

    A. Alien hand syndrome
    B. Klüver–Bucy syndrome
    C. Utilization behaviour
    D. Executive dysfunction
    E. Balint's syndrome

48. **The most probable site of a lesion for the patient described in Question 47 is**

   A. Frontal lobes
   B. Dominant parietal lobe
   C. Occipitoparietal junctions bilaterally
   D. Bilateral amygdala
   E. Corpus callosum

49. **A 32-year-old woman with complex partial seizures is referred to a psychiatrist to exclude psychosis. She experiences olfactory hallucinations and intense anxiety. Which of the following is not correct with regard to complex partial seizures?**

   A. Temporal lobe is the most common site of origin.
   B. Ictal hallucinations are often accompanied by emotional reactions.
   C. Patients are often aware of the unreal nature of the hallucinations.
   D. Irritability is the most common emotional reaction accompanying the aura.
   E. *Déjà vu* is a well-known phenomenon occurring in complex partial seizures.

50. **A 78-year-old woman presents with fluent progressive aphasia with preservation of new learning and orientation. On follow up she is observed to have progressive difficulties in understanding the meaning of words used during normal conversation. She is most likely to have**

   A. Alzheimer's dementia
   B. Semantic dementia
   C. Lewy body dementia
   D. Broca's aphasia
   E. Vitamin B_{12} deficiency

51. **Which of the following can be used to test premorbid IQ in patients with neurological damage?**

   A. National Adult Reading Test
   B. Rivermead Behavioural Memory Test
   C. Weschler's Memory Scale
   D. Mini Mental State Examination
   E. Minnesota Multiphasic Inventory

52. A 55-year-old man with history of long-standing, untreated hypertension is brought to A&E by his wife following 3 hours of 'confusion'. He was repeatedly questioning her and was not able to remember what he was doing 30 minutes ago. He is also unaware of events of the past 2 weeks, despite remembering them until 3 hours ago. Neurological examination is otherwise unremarkable and he has no psychiatric history. The episode resolves by itself within 24 hours. Which of the following is false with regard to his condition?

    A. Immediate memory will be intact.
    B. Anterograde amnesia will be predominant.
    C. Patchy and inconsistent retrograde amnesia will be seen.
    D. Visuospatial and problem-solving functions will be affected.
    E. Rapid recovery occurs in most individuals.

53. Abnormalities in which of the following vascular territories is implicated in the presentation described in Question 52?

    A. Anterior cerebral circulation
    B. Middle cerebral circulation
    C. Posterior cerebral circulation
    D. Cortical venous sinus outflow
    E. Middle meningeal circulation

54. A patient with long-standing, uncontrolled type 2 diabetes presents with anterior spinal artery occlusion. Which of the following sensations carried by the spinal cord is most likely to be affected?

    A. Proprioception
    B. Vibration
    C. Pain
    D. Joint position
    E. Light touch

55. Which of the following structures is a part of cerebellum?

    A. Dentate nucleus
    B. Red nucleus
    C. Substantia nigra
    D. Subthalamic nucleus
    E. Insular cortex

56. Which of the following is true with respect to pseudobulbar palsy?

    A. It is caused by diffuse brain stem damage.
    B. It is often accompanied by flaccid tongue.
    C. Jaw jerk is exaggerated.
    D. It is seen in poliomyelitis.
    E. Frontal release signs are inconsistent with the diagnosis.

57. Lesions of the subthalamic nucleus are associated with

    A. Chorea
    B. Hemiballismus
    C. Tics
    D. Epilepsy
    E. Visual neglect

58. Which of the following neuropsychological tests is primarily used to detect errors in set-shifting capacity?

    A. Tower of London
    B. Rey Osterrieth Complex Figure Test
    C. Wisconsin Card Sorting Test
    D. Word Fluency Test
    E. Letter Cancellation Test

59. A 72-year-old man is afflicted with stroke. He is not able to identify objects with their correct names but is able to demonstrate the usage correctly. When the correct name is given to him, he is able to recognize it correctly. He is suffering from

    A. Motor aphasia
    B. Apraxia
    C. Anomic aphasia
    D. Sensory aphasia
    E. Abulia

60. The blood supply to the hippocampus comes from the

    A. Basilar artery
    B. Anterior communicating artery
    C. Anterior cerebral artery
    D. Anterior choroidal artery
    E. Lenticulostriate arteries

61. In early Alzheimer's disease, widespread loss of nerve cells is most pronounced in which of the following structures?

    A. Layer III of cerebral cortex
    B. Layer IV of entorhinal cortex
    C. Layer I of cerebral cortex
    D. Layer II of entorhinal cortex
    E. Layer IV of cerebral cortex

62. Glutamate-induced excitotoxicity is proposed as a cause of which of the following conditions?

    A. Huntington's disease
    B. Crutzfeld–Jakob disease
    C. Wilson's disease
    D. Korsakoff's syndrome
    E. Weber's syndrome

63. **Which of the following is a feature of occlusion of the right-sided posterior inferior cerebellar artery?**

    A. Left-sided loss of facial pain sensation
    B. Left-sided loss of facial temperature sensation
    C. Loss of pain sensation on the right side of the body
    D. Loss of temperature sensation on the left side of the body
    E. Mydriasis of the right eye

64. **A 65-year-old man presents with memory difficulties and loss of balance. He has significant, new-onset urinary incontinence. CT scan of the brain shows dilated ventricles but no significant widening of sulci. The most likely diagnosis is**

    A. Normal-pressure hydrocephalus
    B. Alzheimer's dementia
    C. Lewy body dementia
    D. Benign intracranial hypertension
    E. Alcoholic dementia

65. **During polysomnographic recording of a patient with sleep disturbances, it is observed that his heart rate and blood pressure are lower than that recorded during normal wakefulness. His muscle tone is also notably low. Which of the following is true with respect to his physiological state?**

    A. Vivid memory of dreams occur at this stage.
    B. If awakened from this stage there will be some degree of confusion.
    C. Penile erection occurs automatically at this stage of sleep.
    D. High cerebral blood flow is seen at this stage.
    E. In adults, 25% of sleeping time is spent in this stage of sleep.

66. **The frequency of alpha waves seen in EEG recordings is**

    A. >13 Hz
    B. 8–12 Hz
    C. 4–8 Hz
    D. 0.5–4 Hz
    E. <0.5 Hz

67. **Diffuse flattening of EEG with low-amplitude theta and delta waves is seen in**

    A. Huntington's disease
    B. Alzheimer's dementia
    C. Hepatic encephalopathy
    D. Delirium tremens
    E. Crutzfeld–Jakob disease

68. **Which of the following functions is mediated by endogenous cannabinoids?**
    A. REM sleep induction
    B. Motor coordination
    C. Peripheral sympathetic modulation
    D. Gut motility
    E. Mediation of intraocular pressure

69. **A 22-year-old man is diagnosed with craniopharyngioma. He is experiencing symptoms due to the tumour pressing upon adjacent brain tissue. Which of the following visual defect is characteristic of this tumour?**
    A. Tunnel vision
    B. Homonymous hemianopia
    C. Binasal hemianopia
    D. Bitemporal hemianopia
    E. Superior quandrantonopia

70. **Priapism is a side-effect associated with which of the following?**
    A. α1 receptor stimulation
    B. α2 receptor stimulation
    C. α1 receptor blockade
    D. α2 receptor blockade
    E. Nicotinic cholinergic stimulation

71. **Metacognitive abilities are proposed to be functions of the frontal lobe. Metacognition refers to**
    A. Planning and sequential execution of motor acts
    B. Ability to reflect on one's own cognitive processes
    C. Problem-solving ability
    D. Initiation and sustainment of motivation
    E. Automatic cognitive processing without selected focus of attention

72. **The 'n-back test' consists of making a response in accordance with a visual or auditory stimulus presented 'n' items before the currently displayed stimulus. This test is widely employed in neuroimaging paradigms primarily to enable engagement of which of the following brain areas?**
    A. Frontal lobes
    B. Occipital lobes
    C. Cerebellum
    D. Hippocampus
    E. Amygdala

73. **Which of the following toxins has been used to simulate a model of Parkinson's disease?**

    A. Ketamine
    B. Methyl phenyl tetrahydropyridine (MPTP)
    C. Methylene dioxy methamphetamine (MDMA)
    D. Vanillyl mandelic acid (VMA)
    E. Hydroxy indole acetic acid (5HIAA)

74. **How many layers are present in the laminar structure of the human cerebral cortex?**

    A. Three
    B. Four
    C. Twelve
    D. Six
    E. Two

75. **Which of the following nuclei of the thalamus is primarily involved in the relay of information for visual processing?**

    A. Supraoptic nucleus
    B. Dorsomedial nucleus
    C. Medial geniculate nucleus
    D. Suprachiasmatic nucleus
    E. Lateral geniculate nucleus

76. **Which of the following cells are the only excitatory neurones in the cerebellum?**

    A. Purkinje cells
    B. Basket cells
    C. Stellate cells
    D. Granule cells
    E. Golgi cells

77. **Which of the following components of cognition is tested by the digit span task?**

    A. Working memory
    B. Implicit memory
    C. Sensory memory
    D. Autobiographic memory
    E. Procedural memory

78. Ataxia can result from cerebellar lesions or posterior column lesions. Though gait disturbances are predominant in both these conditions, which of the following is seen in sensory ataxia but not cerebellar ataxia?

    A. Nystagmus
    B. Dysarthria
    C. Loss of tendon reflexes
    D. Absence of Romberg's sign
    E. Intact joint position sense

79. The ability of neurones to change the connection strength with other neurones underlies the electrophysiological process called long-term potentiation (LTP). Which of the following forms the neurochemical basis of LTP?

    A. Acetylcholine via nicotinic receptors
    B. Substance P
    C. Glutamate via NMDA receptors
    D. Dopamine via D4 receptors
    E. Cannabinoids via CB1 receptors

80. Which of the following is a major dopaminergic site?

    A. Nucleus basalis
    B. Ventral tegmental area
    C. Dorsal raphe nucleus
    D. Spinal interneurones
    E. Locus coeruleus

81. Which of the following brain regions shows a preferential degeneration in Alzheimer's disease?

    A. Nucleus basalis
    B. Ventral tegmental area
    C. Dorsal raphe nucleus
    D. Spinal interneurones
    E. Locus coeruleus

82. Processing of fear conditioning is associated with functions of the

    A. Planum temporale
    B. Heschl's gyrus
    C. Amygdala
    D. Anterior pituitary
    E. Angular gyrus

83. **Which of the following enzymes involved in neurotransmitter synthesis is directly affected by pyridoxine deficiency?**

    A. Glutamate decarboxylase
    B. Acetyl cholinesterase
    C. Dopamine hydroxylase
    D. Tyrosine hydroxylase
    E. Tryptophan hydroxylase

84. **Which of the following brain areas has a relatively permeable blood–tissue interface?**

    A. Anterior pituitary
    B. Hippocampus
    C. Subfornicular organ
    D. Cerebellum
    E. Lateral surface of frontal lobes

85. **Which of the following terms refers to a substance that influences neuronal activity and originates from non-synaptic sites?**

    A. Neurotransmitter
    B. Neurotrophin
    C. Neuromodulator
    D. Second messenger
    E. Neurohormone

86. **Which of the following neurotransmitters act as a physiological antagonist for acetylcholine?**

    A. Serotonin
    B. Substance P
    C. Neurokinin
    D. Norepinephrine
    E. Nicotine

87. **Which of the following is not a ligand-gated ion channel?**

    A. Nicotinic cholinergic receptors
    B. $GABA_A$ receptors
    C. Glycine receptors
    D. NMDA receptors
    E. Muscarinic cholinergic receptors

88. **^{11}C raclopride is a commonly used PET ligand. Which of the following receptors can be identified by ^{11}C raclopride?**

    A. Serotonin receptors
    B. $GABA_A$ receptors
    C. Muscarinic cholinergic recerptors
    D. Postsynaptic dopamine receptors (D2/D3)
    E. Presynaptic dopamine reuptake inhibitor

89. **Leptin is a hormone involved in regulation of adiposity and meal intake. Which of the following structures is the major source of leptin?**

    A. Hypothalamus
    B. Gut epithelium
    C. Hepatocytes in liver
    D. Adipose tissue
    E. Mitochondria-rich muscle fibres

90. **Which of the following substances does not interact with cell membrane receptors and acts directly on nuclear material to produce physiological effects?**

    A. Serotonin
    B. Growth hormone
    C. Norepinephrine
    D. Dopamine
    E. Thyroid hormone

91. **A 77-year-old woman dies of severe pneumonia with sepsis at a care home. She had poor episodic memory for recent events and deteriorating language functions for at least 2 years before her death. The most likely pathology that could be seen in her brain tissue is**

    A. Ballooning of cells with intraneuronal accumulations
    B. Diffuse and neuritic plaques with amyloid deposits in cortex and hippocampus
    C. Diffuse amyloid deposition restricted to blood vessels
    D. Lysosomal accumulations within neuronal cytoplasm
    E. Eosinophilic rod-shaped inclusions of actin filaments

92. **Which of the following receptors, on stimulation, reduces serotonin release?**

    A. 5-HT_{1B}
    B. 5-HT_{1D}
    C. 5-HT_{1A}
    D. 5-HT_{2}
    E. 5-HT_{3}

93. **All of the following are true with respect to dopamine metabolism except**

    A. Monoamine oxidase is the primary metabolic enzyme.
    B. All dopamine from the re-uptake process gets repackaged into presynaptic vesicles.
    C. Catechol-O-methyl transferase is present in cytoplasm of postsynaptic neurones.
    D. Homovanillic acid is a primary metabolite.
    E. Monoamine oxidase type B is more selective for dopamine.

94. **Neuroendocrine abnormalities have been documented in depression and other psychiatric disorders. Which of the following is not a neuroendocrine abnormality seen in depression?**

    A. Blunted growth hormone (GH) response to levodopa
    B. Enhanced growth hormone response to apomorphine
    C. Blunted thyroid-stimulating hormone (TSH) response to thyrotrophin-releasing hormone (TRH)
    D. Failure of exogenous steroid to suppress cortisol
    E. Blunted prolactin release on clomipramine challenge

95. **Event-related potentials (ERP) are records of the brain's electrical activity in response to various stimuli. P300 is an extensively studied ERP in psychiatry. Which of the following is true with respect to P300 abnormalities in schizophrenia?**

    A. P300 is a state rather than a trait marker in schizophrenia.
    B. Schizophrenia with early age of onset shows less pronounced P300 abnormalities.
    C. Reduced P300 amplitude is specific for schizophrenia.
    D. Paranoid subtype is associated with more pronounced P300 abnormalities.
    E. P300 is affected by duration of disease in patients with schizophrenia.

96. **Which of the following tests for intelligence is not influenced by language or formal education?**

    A. Weschler's Adult Intelligence Scale
    B. Stanford–Binet Test
    C. Raven's Progressive Matrices
    D. Weschler's Intelligence Scale For Children
    E. Kaufman Adolescents and Adults Intelligence Test

97. **Neuropeptides such as endorphins are produced from the degradation of a large precursor molecule called pro-opiomelanocortin (POMC). Which of the following hormones is synthesized from the same precursor?**

    A. Thyroxine
    B. Thyroid-stimulating hormone (TSH)
    C. Adrenocorticotrophic hormone (ACTH)
    D. Growth hormone
    E. Antidiuretic hormone (ADH)

98. **All of the following physiological effects are mediated by GABA potentiation except**

    A. Sedation
    B. Working memory
    C. Increase in seizure threshold
    D. Muscle relaxation
    E. Inhibition of memory consolidation

99. Which of the following structures in human brain show morphological differences according to one's sexual orientation?

A. Red nucleus
B. Medial dorsal thalamus
C. Nucleus tractus solitarius
D. Interstitial nucleus of anterior hypothalamus
E. Pineal gland

100. Which of the following proteins is the major component of Lewy bodies seen in Parkinson's disease and Lewy body dementia?

A. Amyloid precursor protein
B. Prion protein
C. Ceruloplasmin
D. Amylin
E. Alpha synuclein

101. Proliferation of large protoplasmic astrocytes results in atypical cells such as Opalski cells and Alzheimer cells. Presence of such astrocytes is a pathological feature of

A. Alzheimer's dementia
B. Fragile-X syndrome
C. Frontotemporal dementia
D. Multiple sclerosis
E. Wilson's disease

102. Which of the following statements regarding the teratogenic effect of alcohol on neuronal development is false?

A. Alcohol induces apoptosis in the fetal brain.
B. Even a single episode of excessive alcohol exposure can be harmful.
C. The most prominent pathological finding in fetal alcohol syndrome is scarring of the thalamus.
D. Facial malformations occur when the exposure is in the first trimester.
E. Thiamine deficiency is the most important mediator of neuronal damage seen in fetal alcohol syndrome.

103. Features of the cauda equina syndrome include all except

A. Asymmetric leg weakness
B. Loss of deep tendon reflex
C. Prominent sphincter dysfunction
D. Low back pain
E. Sensory loss

104. Which of the embryonic germ cell layers give rise to neurones?

A. Neural tube
B. Neural crest
C. Mesoderm
D. Ectoderm
E. Notochord

105. All of the following are features of lesion to the cerebellum except

A. Dysarthria
B. Dysmetria
C. Intentional tremor
D. Ipsilateral hypotonicity
E. Sphincter disturbance

106. Which of the following cranial nerves is purely afferent?

A. Facial nerve
B. Glossopharyngeal nerve
C. Hypoglossal nerve
D. Trochlear nerve
E. Vestibulocochlear nerve

107. The light reflex pathway includes all of the following except

A. Ciliary muscles
B. Edinger–Westphal nucleus
C. Occipital cortex
D. Occulomotor nerve
E. Optic nerve

108. All of the following carry parasympathetic fibres in them except

A. Facial nerve
B. Glossopharyngeal nerve
C. Hypoglossal nerve
D. Oculomotor nerve
E. Vagus nerve

109. Which of the following is a result of parasympathetic activity?

A. Decreased salivation
B. Ejaculation
C. Increased heart rate
D. Relaxation of external anal sphincter
E. Relaxation of the ciliary muscles

110. **The posterior column of the spinal cord is responsible for all of the following except**

   A. Light touch
   B. Proprioception
   C. Tactile localization
   D. Temperature discrimination
   E. Vibration sensation

111. **Which of the following is not a component of the basal ganglia?**

   A. Amygdala
   B. Caudate nucleus
   C. Globus pallidus
   D. Substantia nigra
   E. Subthalamic nucleus

112. **Nystagmus is a recognized feature of all of the following except**

   A. Barbiturate toxicity
   B. Cerebellopontine angle tumours
   C. Horner's syndrome
   D. Multiple sclerosis
   E. Vertibrobasillar artery insufficiency

113. **Which of the following is a feature of normal ageing?**

   A. Preserved immediate memory
   B. Decline in general intelligence measures
   C. Preserved executive abilities such as abstraction
   D. Intact verbal fluency
   E. Intact cognitive processing speed

114. **Which of the following lesions is commonly associated with gelastic (laughing) seizures?**

   A. Hypothalamic tumours
   B. Hippocampal sclerosis
   C. Occipital lesions
   D. Inferior parietal damage
   E. Lesions of corpus callosum

115. **Which of the following is a ligand-gated ion channel?**

   A. Muscarinic receptor
   B. Norepinephrine receptor
   C. Nicotinic receptor
   D. $GABA_B$ receptor
   E. Metabotropic glutamate receptor

116. **A 32-year-old man presents with progressive muscle weakness, cognitive impairment, and involuntary movements of upper limbs and facial muscles. A blood film reveals spiked red blood cells. He is troubled by compulsive behaviour pertaining to order and symmetry. Which of the following conditions is most likely?**

    A. Acanthocytosis
    B. Huntington's chorea
    C. Haemophilia A
    D. Wilson's disease
    E. Progressive supranuclear palsy

117. **The recreational drug LSD exerts its hallucinogenic effect as a partial agonist at which of the following receptors?**

    A. Dopamine D1
    B. Glutamate AMPA
    C. Serotonin 5-HT$_{1A}$
    D. Serotonin 5-HT$_{2A}$
    E. Cannabinoid CB1

118. **Which of the following neurotransmitters is implicated in the neurobiology of addiction and behaviours associated with craving seen in recreational drug users?**

    A. GABA
    B. Dopamine
    C. Substance P
    D. Serotonin
    E. Neurosteroids

119. **Which of the following can be classified as a neurotrophin?**

    A. BDNF
    B. Protein kinase C
    C. Nitric oxide
    D. COMT
    E. Vasopressin

120. **Synthesis of adrenalin from noradrenalin requires which of the following enzymes in a neurone?**

    A. DOPA decarboxylase
    B. Dopamine hydroxylase
    C. Monoamine oxidase
    D. Phenylethanolamine *N*-methyltransferase
    E. Tyrosine hydroxylase

121. **The majority of serotonin in the human body is found in**

    A. Spinal cord
    B. Brain
    C. Gastrointestinal tract
    D. Platelets
    E. Kidneys

122. **Which of the following is a feature of a second messenger?**

    A. They are a class of neurotransmitters.
    B. They are local hormones secreted by neurones into the blood stream.
    C. They are restricted to the peripheral nervous system.
    D. They combine with neurotransmitters in the nucleus.
    E. They mediate the intracellular response to a neurotransmitter.

123. **A 55-year-old man presents to A&E dreading that he has had a stroke. He has a weakness on the right side of his face with drooling of saliva from the right corner of his mouth. On examination he is not able to close his right eye fully and cannot hold air against his right cheek. When attempting a wrinkle, the right eyebrow appears sluggish. He is not able to whistle properly. He has normal tone and power in all four limbs. Which of the following clinical signs can be expected?**

    A. Bell's phenomenon
    B. Nystagmus
    C. Miosis of left eye
    D. Plantar extensor
    E. Mydriasis of right eye

124. **Regarding the serotonin (5-HT) system in the brain, which of the follow statements is false?**

    A. Serotonergic cells are localized in the raphe nuclei.
    B. Serotonergic cells project to virtually all areas of the brain.
    C. 5-HT receptors are mostly ionotropic.
    D. Serotonin does not cross the blood–brain barrier.
    E. Serotonin is synthesized from tryptophan.

125. **Prion protein PrP^C is seen in normal cells. Pathological changes in this protein can lead to neurodegenerative changes seen in Cruetzfeldt–Jakob disease. Which of the following explanations in most likely for the pathological variation?**

    A. The pathological protein has a different amino-acid sequence compared to the normal protein.
    B. The pathological protein differs from normal protein in the quantity produced but not in the quality.
    C. The pathological protein is structurally different from normal protein.
    D. The pathological protein is coded by a genetically transmitted mutant DNA.
    E. The pathological protein suppresses the immune system.

126. **Which of the following brain regions is involved in the regulation of arousal and sleep–wake cycle?**

    A. Amygdala
    B. Cingulate cortex
    C. Hippocampus
    D. Reticular system
    E. Ventral striatum

127. **The resting membrane potential of a neurone is estimated to be approximately**

    A. +70 mV
    B. +90 mV
    C. 0 mV
    D. −30 V
    E. −70 mV

128. **Which of the following statements with respect to the neurotransmitter glycine is correct?**

    A. It is primarily an excitatory neurotransmitter.
    B. It acts via GABAA receptors.
    C. It is associated with idiopathic epilepsy.
    D. It facilitates chloride ion entry into neurones.
    E. It is most abundant in dorsolateral prefrontal cortex.

129. **Direct measurement of cerebral glucose metabolism is possible using which of the following methods?**

    A. Single photon emission computed tomography
    B. Computed tomography with radiocontrast
    C. Positron emission tomography
    D. Functional magnetic resonance imaging
    E. Magnetoencephalography

130. **A nocturnal surge in the level of growth hormones is observed during which of the following stages of sleep?**

    A. REM sleep
    B. Stage 1 and 2 NREM sleep
    C. Stage 3 and 4 NREM sleep
    D. All stages of sleep
    E. Upon awakening

131. A 15-year-old boy is brought to paediatric A&E by his parents. He complains of severe headache and vomits while waiting to be seen. He gives a history of polyuria and confusion with visual field defects. On examination he appears to be significantly shorter than average height for his age. He does not have signs of meningitis. His past medical history and family history reveals no additional clues to his presentation. He denies using drugs. Which of the following investigations may help in clinching the diagnosis?

    A. CSF analysis
    B. Electroencephalogram
    C. CT brain scan
    D. Neuropsychological testing
    E. Urine drug screen

132. Which of the following structures may be causally related to the presentation in Question 131?

    A. Alar plate
    B. C cells of thyroid
    C. Isthumus of thyroid
    D. Neural tube
    E. Rathke's pouch

133. A 45-year-old man presents with sudden onset, uncontrolled, wide flinging movements of his left arm and leg. He is a known diabetic and has not been taking his antihypertensive medications for the last 2 months. He is cognitively intact. Which of the following is the most likely site of a lesion?

    A. Left cerebellum
    B. Left putamen
    C. Right internal capsule
    D. Right subthalamic nucleus
    E. Right thalamus

134. Phineas Gage is a celebrated case in neuropsychiatry. This 25-year-old railroad foreman sustained an extraordinary brain injury after which he had a significant change in his personality characterized by childishness, stubborn, and obstinate behaviour with frequent use of profanities. Which of the following brain regions was damaged significantly to result in this presentation?

    A. Inferior parietal cortex
    B. Superior temporal cortex
    C. Orbitofrontal cortex
    D. Hippocampus
    E. Hypothalamus

135. A 60-year-old man presents with a 4-week history of right foot pain and sensory loss. The GP prescribes an analgesic and makes a referral to a neurologist. While awaiting the specialist appointment, the patient develops left-sided wrist drop and weakness of right hand grip. He does not have any autonomic disturbances and appears to be cognitively intact. The most common cause of the above presentation is

    A. Diabetes mellitus
    B. Periarteritis nodosa
    C. Sarcoidosis
    D. Leprosy
    E. Temporal arteritis

136. A neuropsychologist administers a test to a 21-year-old man with a change in personality related to brain damage. The patient is asked to name the colour of a word while ignoring the actual word. What test is being administered?

    A. Wisconsin Card Sorting Test
    B. Benton Visuomotor Test
    C. Rorschach's Test
    D. Continuous Performance Test
    E. Stroop Test

137. Which of the following is the rate-limiting enzyme in the synthesis of dopamine?

    A. Tyrosine hydroxylase
    B. DOPA decarboxylase
    C. Dopamine hydroxylase
    D. Monoamine oxydase
    E. Catechol-O-methyl transferase

138. A 55-year-old patient presents with bilateral hand tremors that worsen with stress. Which of the following features of the tremor is suggestive of benign essential tremor rather than Parkinsonism?

    A. Tremor is increased by alcohol
    B. Tremor is reduced by action
    C. Tremor is absent at rest
    D. Frequency of the tremor is 4–6 cycles per second
    E. The amplitude of the tremor is large

139. A 50-year-old woman, being treated for depression as an outpatient, presents to A&E with acute-onset, severe headache. She describes this as the 'worst headache' she has ever had in her life. She insists on switching off the lights in the examination cubicle. Her blood pressure is 150/90 mmHg. When asked to get up from the examination couch, she complains of neck stiffness. An emergency CT scan is normal. The next most appropriate step is

A. Change her antidepressant
B. Obtain MRI scan
C. Obtain urine drug screen
D. Prepare for lumbar puncture
E. Prescribe haloperidol 2.5 mg only

140. A 68-year-old woman has long-standing hypertension. She is diagnosed to have somatization disorder by her GP and is prescribed venlafaxine 225 mg/day. Unfortunately she develops a cerebrovascular accident. While being treated for stroke at the acute neurology unit, she starts having severe, 'gruesome' pain on her left side of the body. The pain has an intense, scalding quality. The most likely site of infarct is

A. Cerebellum
B. Cerebello pontine junction
C. Thalamus
D. Hippocampus
E. Internal capsule

1.A. The answer is Parkinson's disease. Bradykinesia or hypokinesia is a motor feature of Parkinson's disease. Dysarthria is a deficit in the motor aspect of speech. It is usually secondary to a motor neurological deficit. Dysarthria can affect not only articulation, but also phonation, breathing, or prosody (emotional tone) of speech. Total loss of ability to articulate is called anarthria, whereas dysarthria usually involves the distortion of consonant sounds. The Mayo Clinic classification of dysarthria divides dysarthria into six basic types, each one corresponding to a predominant motor disorder: flaccid (lower motor neurone disorders), spastic (upper motor neurone disorders), ataxic (cerebellar lesions), hypokinetic (parkinsonian), hyperkinetic (choreiform/tic disorders), and mixed. Mixed dysarthrias are seen in conditions with multiple motor lesions, for example mixed spastic–ataxia of multiple sclerosis or mixed spastic–flaccidity of amyotrophic lateral sclerosis. Speech therapy may be of substantial benefit to many dysarthric patients.

Cummings JL and Mega MS. *Neuropsychiatry and Behavioural Neuroscience.* Oxford University Press, 2003, p. 74.
Bradley WG, Daroff RB, Fenichel G, and Jankovic J. *Neurology in Clinical Practice: Principles of Diagnosis and Management,* 4th edn. Butterworth-Heinemann, 2003, p. 162.

2.D. Testing a person's speech is usually done in three steps. The first step is to test for the fluency of speech. Non-fluent output is characterized by a paucity of verbal output (usually 10–50 words per minute), whereas fluent aphasics have a normal or even exaggerated verbal output (up to 200 words or more per minute). Lesions of the motor (Broca's) area produce a non-fluent aphasia. Assessment of language comprehension is the second step. Patients with focal lesions limited to the left frontal lobe (Broca's area) will have preserved comprehension (Broca's and transcortical motor aphasia). Patients with left posterior temporal or parietal involvement will show impaired comprehension (Wernicke's, global, transcortical sensory, and isolation aphasias). The third step is to evaluate repetition. Transcortical aphasias usually have an intact repetition. Patients with Broca's, Wernicke's, or conduction aphasia typically show impaired repetition. In conduction aphasia, speech is fluent (as in Wernicke's aphasia) but comprehension is intact (unlike Wernicke's aphasia).

Cummings JL and Mega MS. *Neuropsychiatry and Behavioural Neuroscience.* Oxford University Press, 2003, p. 74.

3. A. Transcortical sensory aphasia is similar to Wernicke,s aphasia but is distinguished by the retained ability to repeat. Lesions causing transcortical aphasias do not disrupt the perisylvian language circuit from Wernicke's area through the arcuate fasciculus to Broca's area. Instead, they interrupt connections from other cortical centres into the language circuit (hence the name transcortical). These areas include the dominant angular gyrus, posterior middle temporal gyrus, and periventricular white matter pathways of the temporal isthmus underlying these cortical areas. When this results from involvement of the angular gyrus, it is frequently accompanied by Gerstmann's syndrome, constructional apraxia, and other evidence of the angular gyrus syndrome.

Cummings JL and Mega MS. *Neuropsychiatry and Behavioural Neuroscience.* Oxford University Press, 2003, p. 79.

4. C. Paragrammatism is seen in Wernicke's aphasia. Speech is characterized by being empty of meaning, containing verbal paraphasias, neologisms, and jargon productions. Most patients with Wernicke's aphasia have no elementary motor or sensory deficits. A right homonymous hemianopia may be present. Patients may be unaware of the deficit and may present with paranoia, as they do not realize why others do not understand them. The presence of paragrammatism may be difficult to distinguish from formal thought disorder in schizophrenia. In contrast, Broca's aphasia shows agrammatism. In this case, the speech pattern is non-fluent; on examination, the patient speaks hesitantly, often producing the principal, meaning-containing nouns and verbs but omitting small grammatical words and morphemes. This pattern is called agrammatism or telegraphic speech, for example: 'I go home' or 'wife here morning'. Reading is often impaired in Broca's aphasia despite preserved auditory comprehension. Broca's aphasia is associated with right hemiparesis, hemisensory loss, and apraxia of the non-paralysed left limbs. Due to the awareness of the deficit, patients with Broca's aphasia may be more prone to depression. Pure word deafness is a syndrome of isolated loss of auditory comprehension and repetition, without any abnormality of speech, naming, reading, or writing. It is caused by bilateral, or sometimes a unilateral, lesion, isolating Wernicke's area from input from both Heschl's gyri. A lesion representing most of the territory of the left middle cerebral (not posterior circulation) artery leads to a global aphasia.

Bradley WG, Daroff RB, Fenichel G, and Jankovic J. *Neurology in Clinical Practice: Principles of Diagnosis and Management*, 4th edn. Butterworth-Heinemann, 2003, p. 144.

5. E. Pure alexia without agraphia is associated with left posterior cerebral artery stroke, with infarction of the medial occipital lobe, often the splenium of the corpus callosum, and often the medial temporal lobe. Alexia is the acquired inability to read. Patients with alexia without agraphia can write but cannot read their own writing. Alexia with agraphia is sometimes called acquired illiteracy. Alexia with agraphia is seen in angular gyrus lesions and is associated with Gerstmann's syndrome. It is seen in stroke of the angular branch of the middle cerebral artery. Transcortical aphasias are analogues to the syndromes of global, Broca's, and Wernicke's aphasias, with intact repetition. Lesions producing transcortical aphasias disrupt connections from other cortical centres into the language circuit. Lesions to the arcuate fasciculus (usually in either the superior temporal or inferior parietal regions) present with conduction aphasia.

Bradley WG, Daroff RB, Fenichel G, and Jankovic J. *Neurology in Clinical Practice: Principles of Diagnosis and Management*, 4th edn. Butterworth-Heinemann, 2003, pp. 144–146.

6. D. Inferior olivary lesions lead to appendicular ataxia which can be tested using the finger–nose test. The inferior olivary nucleus serves motor coordination via projecting climbing fibres to the cerebellum. Isolated lesions of superior colliculus result in defective visual saccades. Subtle auditory defects are noted in similar lesions of the inferior colliculus. Pyramidal decussation carries corticospinal fibres; damage to the corticospinal fibres rostral to (above) the pyramidal decussation results in contralateral motor deficits, while lesions below the decussation result in ipsilateral deficits. Thalamic damage often results in sensory deficit syndromes.

Ruigrok TJ. Cerebellar nuclei: the olivary connection. *Progress in Brain Research* 1997; **114**: 167–192.

7. E. Echolalia is the phenomenon where the patient repeats words or phrases said by the examiner; palilalia is the phenomenon where the patient repeats words or phrases that he has uttered himself. In patients who develop both phenomena, echolalia precedes the onset of palilalia. Common causes of echolalia include the transcortical aphasias and disorders that affect the basal ganglia–frontal circuit. Echolalia could be due to a frontal executive deficit, leading to failure of environmental autonomy and resulting in echoing of perceived environmental stimuli. Palilalia should be distinguished from stuttering and logoclonia (repetition of the final syllable of spoken words). Echolalia may be observed as part of speech disturbances in catatonic states.

Cummings JL and Mega MS. *Neuropsychiatry and Behavioural Neuroscience.* Oxford University Press, 2003, p. 90.

8. E. Orientation is a measure of cognitive function. NPI is used for the assessment of thought disturbance, perceptual disturbances, affect, abulia, agitation/aggression, disinhibition, appetite disturbance, sleeping pattern, and aberrant motor activity in patients with dementia/cognitive deficits. It does not test cognitive functions such as memory or orientation.

Goldstein MA. and Silverman ME. Neuropsychiatric assessment. *Psychiatric Clinics of North America* 2005; **28**: 511–515.

9. D. Hemispheric dominance is clinically inferred by handedness. It is a peripheral indicator of cerebral hemispheric language lateralization. Handedness is now considered to exist as a continuum, from extreme unilateral hand dominance on one end to ambidexterity on the other. In this respect, the Edinburgh Handedness Inventory is a semiquantitative measurement of handedness. It is thought that at least 90% of the human population is right-handed. Of these, 95% are left-hemisphere dominant. Approximately 10% of the human population is left-handed and of these at least 60% are left-hemisphere dominant. Left-handers are more likely to have bilateral language representation.

Goldstein MA. and Silverman ME. Neuropsychiatric assessment. *Psychiatric Clinics of North America* 2005; **28**: 511–515.

10. D. This test is called the trail making test. It is not only a test of attention, but it also tests visuomotor tracking and cognitive flexibility (part B). Trail making test A requires the subject to connect numbered dots. Trail making test B requires the subject to connect alternating alphabets and numbers. This tests the ability to shift mental sets and hence to some extent corresponds to executive functioning. This has been shown to be sensitive to change in patients with progressive cognitive decline (e.g. dementia). Patients with traumatic brain injury perform slower on trail making tests.

Lezak MD *et al.*, eds. *Neuropsychological Assessment*, 4th edn. Oxford University Press, 2004, pp. 372–374.

11. D. Medial temporal cortex is not supplied by the anterior communicating artery; it is supplied by the posterior cerebral artery. The anterior communicating artery supplies the basal forebrain and striatum. Wernicke–Korsakoff syndrome is usually associated with nutritional causes, where the thalamic nuclei (especially dorsal medial thalamus) are involved, leading to anterograde amnesia and confabulation. Herpes simplex encephalitis (HSE) is another cause of anterograde amnesia where anterior temporal lobes are often involved. Whether amnesia is predominantly verbal or non-verbal is determined by the side of lesion and the cerebral dominance. In CJD (Creutzfeldt–Jacob disease) diffuse cortical damage occurs. Amnesia of complex partial seizures is related to recurrent hippocampal damage and sclerosis.

Goldstein MA. and Silverman ME. Neuropsychiatric assessment. *Psychiatric Clinics of North America* 2005; **28**: 526.

12. D. Balint's syndrome consist of a triad of oculomotor apraxia (deficits in the orderly visuomotor scanning of the environment), optic ataxia (inaccurate manual reaching toward visual targets), and simultanagnosia. Pathologically, Balint's syndrome is produced by bilateral parieto-occipital lesions. Simultanagnosia is the inability to integrate visual information in the centre of gaze with more peripheral information. The patient gets stuck on the detail that falls in the centre of gaze without scanning the visual environment for additional information. They typically 'miss the forest for the trees.' This leads to a significant disturbance in object identification. A patient with Balint's syndrome when shown a table lamp and asked to name the object may look at its circular base and call it an ash tray!

Kasper DL *et al.*, eds. *Harrison's Principles of Internal Medicine*, 16th edn. McGraw-Hill, 2005, p. 150.

13. C. Dysarthria is not a feature of Gerstmann's syndrome. Full Gerstmann's syndrome, though rarely reported, consists of left–right disorientation, finger agnosia, dysgraphia, and dyscalculia. The lesion is mostly attributed to a dominant parietal lobe dysfunction. When all the components are present the syndrome reliably localizes to the dominant angular gyrus. Gerstmann himself thought that the inability to calculate was because of the fact that children learnt to count with their fingers and the dysgraphia was due to problems with differential finger movements—both being secondary to finger agnosia. Gerstmann noted that the greatest trouble in finger agnostics was with distinguishing second, third, and fourth fingers. Screening for full Gerstmann's syndrome should be performed on patients who show any single component.

Cummings JL and Mega MS. *Neuropsychiatry and Behavioural Neuroscience*. Oxford University Press, 2003, p. 87.

14. D. Anton's syndrome features blindness and denial of blindness, that is the patient is blind but denies sightlessness. The syndrome is most commonly associated with bilateral lesions of the occipital cortex. Blind sight is a paradoxical syndrome seen in patients with cortical blindness. It is the ability of the person to orient towards visual stimuli while there is no conscious visual perception. This is due to the fact that 20 to 30% of fibres of the optic tract are directed to non-geniculate destinations, such as the superior colliculi and pretectal region of the brainstem. It is thought that some visual processing occurs in this non-geniculate system. This phenomenon is not demonstrable if the blindness is the result of pregeniculate lesions. Geschwind's syndrome refers to personality changes proposed to be due to disconnection of brain areas noted in those with temporal lobe epilepsy. The Charcot–Wilbrand syndrome, or irreminiscence, is characterized by the inability to generate an internal mental image or revisualize (imagine) an object. The patients have more difficulty in generating objects through drawing than in copying model figures. It is usually secondary to bilateral parietal lobe lesions. Central achromatopsia refers to loss of colour vision due to occipital lobe lesions.

Cummings JL and Mega MS. *Neuropsychiatry and Behavioural Neuroscience*. Oxford University Press, 2003, p. 123.

15. A. Ideational apraxia (IDA) is an inability to correctly sequence a series of acts that lead to a goal. Asking the patient to carry out a multistep, sequential task, such as preparing a sandwich for work, is a good test of IDA. It is most often associated with degenerative dementia and delirium. Ideomotor apraxia is probably the most common type of apraxia. Patients with ideomotor apraxia make spatial and temporal errors when performing learned, skilled movements including pantomimes, imitations, and using actual objects. When pantomiming the use of a screwdriver, patients with ideomotor apraxia may rotate their arm at the shoulder and fix their elbow. In right-handed individuals ideomotor apraxia is almost always associated with left-hemisphere lesions. A variety of structures, including the corpus callosum, the inferior parietal lobe, and the premotor areas, may be involved. Patients with ideomotor apraxia can imitate actions of others (using tools/objects) but have difficulty pantomiming (in the absence of tools/objects). In patients with conduction apraxia, imitation is worse than pantomiming. The site of the lesion has not been localized (unlike conduction aphasia). Patients with conceptual apraxia make tool-selection errors.

Ropper AH and Brown RH, eds. *Adam and Victor's Principles of Neurology*, 8th edn. McGraw-Hill, 2005, p. 402.

16. D. Limb-kinetic apraxia most often occurs in the limb contralateral to a hemispheric lesion, usually to the premotor cortex. Patients with limb-kinetic apraxia demonstrate a loss of deftness and ability to make finely graded, precise, independent finger movements. These subjects will not be able to use a pincher grasp to pick up a penny. They will have trouble rotating a coin between the thumb, middle finger, and little finger.

Ropper AH and Brown RH, eds. *Adam and Victor's Principles of Neurology*, 8th edn. McGraw-Hill, 2005, p. 402.

17. A. The term agnosia was originally introduced by Freud. In general, patients with agnosia have clinical feature of impaired recognition of sensory stimuli despite normal sensory pathways. Agnosia represents a disorder of higher-order sensory processing. There is an impaired ability to recognize the nature or meaning of sensory stimuli. This is usually modality specific. There are two basic categories of agnosia. Apperceptive agnosia involves impaired generation of the minimal integrated percept necessary for meaningful recognition. This defect, leads to the formation of an inadequate minimal object recognition unit (i.e. the minimum information required to meaningfully interpret the percept). For example, a "pencil" is initially perceived as—"long, thin, pointed at one end, etc", before a meaning ("it is a pencil—it is used to write") is attributed to the percept. Patients are unable to distinguish visual shapes and so have trouble recognizing, copying, or discriminating between different visual stimuli. Associative agnosia involves defective association of meaning with percepts. The defect is in associating a correctly perceived percept with its meaning. Patients can describe visual scenes and classes of objects but still fail to recognize them. Patients suffering from associative agnosia are still able to reproduce an image through copying. Anosognosia refers to being unaware of a neurological state/illness. Abulia refers to loss of drive or motivation seen in cingulate lesions.

Goldstein MA. and Silverman ME. Neuropsychiatric assessment. *Psychiatric Clinics of North America* 2005; **28**: 530.

18. B. Since this person has a difficulty in recognizing faces, he is suffering from prosopagnosia. In this situation, he can differentiate between faces. So, the defect is probably at a step after the formation of the minimal recognition unit (described in the previous question), but at the step where the percept (in this case the face) is associated with a meaning ('whose face it is'). So this patient is most probably suffering from associative prosopagnosia.

Goldstein MA. and Silverman ME. Neuropsychiatric assessment. *Psychiatric Clinics of North America* 2005; **28**: 534.

19. C. Memories of specific experiences formed in specific contexts are called episodic, for example the meal one had 3 weeks ago at a restaurant. Episodic memory is explicit, that is it is consciously acquired (we know how and where we acquire it) and declarative, that is it can be consciously recalled. Episodic memory depends largely on the integrity of the medial temporal lobe, but there are other structures that are involved in episodic memory. These include the frontal lobe, basal forebrain, retrosplenial cortex, presubiculum, fornix, mammillary bodies, mammillothalamic tract, anterior nucleus of the thalamus, etc. Damage to any one of these structures can result in deficits in episodic memory. Hence episodic memory loss cannot be said to be characteristic of a medial temporal lesion. Episodic memory impairment could manifest as anterograde or retrograde amnesia. Anterograde amnesia refers to impairment in new memory formation and retrograde amnesia refers to the loss of previously acquired memories. Episodic memory applies to both personal and public events. In most dementias, semantic memory loss occurs at later stages than episodic memory loss.

Budson AE and Price BH. Memory dysfunction. *New England Journal of Medicine* 2005; **352**: 692–699.

20. C. Semantic memory describes memories for general information which is unrelated to other information, for example dates in history, the colour of our national flag, or the characteristics of different species of dinosaurs (encyclopaedic facts). Semantic memory is explicit and declarative (see explanation to the previous question). In the most general sense, semantic memory refers to all of our knowledge of the world; however, semantic memory is more usually tested in the context of naming and categorization tasks. It is localized to the inferior lateral temporal lobes. The frontal lobes are responsible for providing information to, and retrieving information out of, the semantic memory banks.

Budson AE and Price BH. Memory dysfunction. *New England Journal of Medicine* 2005; **352**: 692–699.

21. E. The woman described in the question probably suffers from dissociative amnesia, in this case precipitated by the stress of separation. Systematized amnesia is the loss of memory for a certain category of information such as material relating to one's family or a particular person. In this case, her boy friend. Localized amnesia is the condition where the individual fails to recall events that occurred during a circumscribed period of time. In selective amnesia the person can recall some but not all events during a circumscribed period of time. Generalized amnesia is characterized by a failure to recall all of a person's past life. There may be dissociation between explicit and implicit memory, for example the person may retain all his learned skills, but completely forget who he is or his past (a la Jason Bourne in the Bourne trilogy). Continuous amnesia is a condition featuring an inability to recall events subsequent to a specific time up to and including the present.

Cummings JL and Mega MS. *Neuropsychiatry and Behavioural Neuroscience.* Oxford University Press, 2003, p. 334.

22. D.   Working memory describes the ability to temporarily hold information in mind and manipulate it as required by circumstances, for example doing mental arithmetic. It may be phonological, such as keeping a phone number in mind for as long as it takes to dial or visuospatial, such as following a mental map while cycling to work. Baddeley described a central executive system in working memory, which is central to manipulation of the data held in the 'phonological loop' or the 'visuospatial sketchpad'. In short, working memory is what allows us to mentally add up the cost of the number of pints of lager we had at the pub, subtract the total from the value of the money we give the bar tender, and calculate the change that is due to us. Prefrontal cortex is the most important structure for working memory, due to the extensive role played by the central executive; other structures involved include posterior parietal cortices. Disturbances of working memory can result in anterograde disturbances to other systems of memory as well, because intact working memory is generally required for the encoding of information. Episodic memory may be particularly affected.

Budson AE and Price BH. Memory dysfunction. *New England Journal of Medicine* 2005; **352**: 692–699.

23. E.   Procedural memory describes the ability to learn and perform tasks without conscious thought. This is disturbed in conditions that involve subcortical basal ganglia structures such as Parkinson's disease, Huntington's disease, progressive supranuclear palsy, and olivopontocerebellar degeneration. Procedural memory deficits may also be found in depression and OCD. In conditions such as Alzheimer's disease, mild cognitive impairment, Lewy body dementia, vascular dementia, the frontal variant of frontotemporal dementia, encephalitis, Korsakoff's syndrome, traumatic brain injury, hypoxic–ischaemic brain injury (including cardiac bypass surgeries), temporal lobe surgery, seizures, vitamin B_{12} deficiency, hypoglycaemia, transient global amnesia, and multiple sclerosis, episodic memory is more likely to be impaired. Mood, anxiety, and psychotic disorders may also show episodic memory disturbances. Finally, episodic memory impairment may be a side-effect of treatment with anticholinergic drugs and ECT. Semantic memory may be disturbed in conditions such as Alzheimer's disease, the temporal variant of frontotemporal dementia, traumatic brain injury, and encephalitis. Working memory is disturbed in most of the conditions listed above. Working memory is also impaired in anxiety, depression, schizophrenia, OCD, ADHD, other psychiatric states, and medications. Finally, impairments in working memory occur as part of normal ageing.

Budson AE and Price BH. Memory dysfunction. *New England Journal of Medicine* 2005; **352**: 692–699.

24. E.   The condition described is Wernicke–Korsakoff syndrome. Although the common cause for the syndrome is malnutrition secondary to alcohol use, a number of other conditions including hyperemesis during pregnancy, gastrectomy, pyloric stenosis, etc. are associated. In addition to difficulty learning new information, patients with Korsakoff's syndrome usually have a retrograde amnesia which could extend back up to several years prior to the onset of the syndrome. Patients usually remain amnesic for 1–3 months after onset and then begin to recover gradually over a 10-month period; 25% recover completely and 25% have no demonstrable recovery. CT scan may reveal bilateral hypodense areas in the medial thalamus in patients with acute Wernicke's encephalopathy, and mamillary body atrophy may be demonstrated by MRI in some patients with chronic Korsakoff's syndrome. Confabulation is common during the early phases of Korsakoff's syndrome but is unusual in the chronic phase of the condition. Administration of thiamine during the acute Wernicke's phase may prevent emergence of Korsakoff's syndrome. Once the memory defect is established, however, thiamine has little effect except to prevent further deterioration.

Cummings JL and Mega MS. *Neuropsychiatry and Behavioural Neuroscience.* Oxford University Press, 2003, p. 100.

25. A.   There are several clinical indicators that predict severity of a head injury. They include duration of retrograde amnesia, the depth of unconsciousness as assessed by the worst score on the Glasgow Coma Scale (GCS), the duration of coma, neurological evidence of cerebral injury, using an MRI or EEG, and the duration of post-traumatic amnesia. Of these, the least useful clinical indicator is the duration of retrograde amnesia. Duration of post-traumatic amnesia is the best marker of outcome. Patients with a post-traumatic amnesia of less than 1 week will have minimal disability, while duration of more than 1 month is suggestive of enduring and significant disability. Other predictors of a bad outcome include previous head injury, older age, *APOE e4* status, and alcohol dependence. Head injury can be classified as mild wherein a GCS score of 13 to 15 is likely to be associated with only a short duration of loss of consciousness (less than 20 minutes) and a short post-traumatic amnesia (less than 24 hours). In moderate head injury, GCS score 9 to 12 is likely to be associated with loss of consciousness of more than a few minutes but less than 24 hours and a post-traumatic amnesia of more than 1 day but less than 1 week. In severe head injury, a GCS score 3 to 8 is likely to be associated with a loss of consciousness of more than 1 day or a post-traumatic amnesia of more than 1 week.

Gelder MG *et al.*, eds. *New Oxford Textbook of Psychiatry.* Oxford University Press, 2000, p. 441.

26. B.   The term post-concussion syndrome (PCS) is used to describe a cluster of symptoms that results in severe disability following mild head injury. There is no consistent relationship between the prevalence of PCS and the severity of head injury. Sometimes a similar constellation of symptoms may be seen in moderate and severe injury, where it is more likely to be attributed to the actual brain damage. Symptoms are usually vague, but early symptoms may include neurological complaints such as diplopia, dizziness, etc. Additional symptoms include cognitive impairment, fatigue, anxiety, depression, and irritability. In general, most neurological symptoms will have resolved by 2 to 6 months. Several observations support an organic basis, for example diffuse microscopic axonal injury on post mortem, macroscopic brain lesions evident in 8–10% of individuals on CT scan, subtle abnormalities on EEG, etc. Psychosocial factors play a part in the syndrome, especially in those lasting longer than 1 year. This is greatest in those with very mild head injuries and very chronic symptoms. There is an association between severity of post-concussion symptoms and seeking compensation, but very few improve even after the compensation.

King NS. The post concussion syndrome: Clarity amid the controversy? *British Journal of Psychiatry* 2003; **183**: 276–278.

27. E.   Anticonvulsants are not indicated at this point in time, especially since the patient has no symptoms suggestive of seizures. About 2 to 5% of all patients with mild, closed head injury tend to develop long-term seizure disorder. This rises to about 10 to 20% in patients with severe, closed head injury. A higher incidence of seizures has been seen in patients with depressed skull fractures (15%), haematomas (30%), and penetrating brain wounds (50%). Early seizures, within the first week, are relatively benign and are only weak predictors of later epilepsy. This patient has a mild, closed injury, and he is at a low risk for developing seizures, despite positive family history. Randomized controlled studies have shown that the use of anticonvulsants does not prevent the development of post-traumatic epilepsy beyond the first week after injury. There is a limited role for genetic predisposition in developing post-traumatic epilepsy. Those with the *ApoE-ε4* allele may be at higher risk for post-traumatic epilepsy.

Frey LC. Epidemiology of posttraumatic epilepsy: a critical review. *Epilepsia* 2003; **44** (s10): 11–17.

28. D. This patient is most probably suffering from multiple sclerosis. The lifetime prevalence of major depression in multiple sclerosis (MS) is around 50%. It is three to 10 times the rate in the general population. Suicidal intent occurs in up to 30% of MS patients. This is linked to the presence and severity of depression and degree of social isolation. Suicide rates in MS patients are up to seven times higher than rates in the general population. Depression and suicide rates are higher in MS than in most other neurologic disorders. In MS patients, the lifetime prevalence of bipolar affective disorder is twice the prevalence in the general population. Pathological laughing and crying is a syndrome that presents with inappropriate laughter without associated happiness and inappropriate tears without associated sadness. Approximately 10% of MS patients are affected, with varying degrees of severity. ECT is generally well tolerated by patients with MS, but carries a risk of neurological relapse and exacerbation of the illness.

Feinstein A. The neuropsychiatry of multiple sclerosis. *Canadian Journal of Psychiatry* 2004; **49**: 157–163.

29. C. Around 50% of patients with MS have cognitive deficits. Aphasia, apraxia, and agnosia, which are characteristic of predominantly cortical diseases, are generally absent in MS, where pathology is largely confined to subcortical white matter. Although patients with long-lasting and advanced physical disability may also have severe cognitive impairment, the correlation between cognitive dysfunction and disease characteristics (type and duration of MS) is usually weak or modest. Cognitive deficits are also independent of mood symptoms in MS. Deficits in working, semantic, and episodic memories have been reported. MS patients have difficulty both in acquiring and in retrieving information (although performance on recognition tests is better than recall). Procedural memory is usually unaffected. Impaired attention and slowness of thinking is another feature of MS. Frontal lobe deficits may take the form of deficits in conceptualization and abstract thinking. At least one study has shown that donepezil is effective in improving cognitive deficits in MS.

Jefferies K. The neuropsychiatry of multiple sclerosis. *Advances in Psychiatric Treatment* 2006; **12**: 214–220.

30. D. Pathological laughter and crying is a symptom seen in MS, where approximately 10% of MS patients are affected, with varying degrees of severity. This is similar to descriptions of the pseudobulbar affect, although this symptom can be present without pseudobulbar palsy. Patients are more likely to have frontally mediated cognitive deficits. Commonly used scales to identify and characterize this syndrome include the Pathological Laughter and Crying Scale and the Centre for Neurologic Study–Lability Scale. The most common differential diagnosis is a mood disorder, but patients with pathological crying exhibit the emotional display in the absence of a pervasive and sustained elation or depressed mood. But when mood disorder and pathological laughter and crying coexist, differentiation can be very difficult. TCAs and SSRIs have been found to be effective in the treatment even if no depression is noted.

Parvizi J, Arciniegas DB, Bernardini GL et al. Diagnosis and management of pathological laughter and crying. *Mayo Clinic Proceedings* 2006; **81**: 1482–1486.

31. B. Epilepsy is a common disorder, affecting approximately 1% of the population and may involve individuals of any age. Seizures are convulsions that may be produced by a wide variety of events, including alcohol and drug withdrawal syndromes, hypoglycaemia, transient cerebral anoxia, and epileptic syndromes. Epilepsies are characterized by recurrent seizures and their classification is based on seizure type, age of onset, intellectual development, findings on neurological examination, and results of neuroimaging studies. Seizures are broadly classified into partial and general forms. Partial seizures are further divided into simple and complex. In simple partial seizures consciousness is preserved; complex seizures are characterized by disturbances in consciousness. Partial seizures pertain to one half or one particular area of the brain. Generalized seizures involve both hemispheres from the beginning of the seizure but, at times, they may be secondary to spread from a partial seizure. Tonic–clonic seizures and absence seizures are examples of primary generalized seizures. They are usually associated with a loss of conscious awareness.

Ropper AH and Brown RH, eds. *Adam and Victor's Principles of Neurology*, 8th edn. McGraw-Hill, 2005, p. 275.

32. D. Left-sided foci are associated with an increased risk of depression and right-sided foci with an increased risk of mania. Mood disorders are the most common type of psychopathology encountered in patients with epilepsy. Prevalence rates of depression range from 30 to 50% in patients with epilepsy. With intractable disorders, up to 60% have lifetime histories of depressive syndromes. In contrast to the incidence of depression in epilepsy, the incidence of mania and bipolar disorder are at normal or near-normal levels. Some retrospective chart reviews state a lifetime prevalence of 20%. The incidence of suicide in epilepsy patients is five to 10-fold greater than in the general population. In those with temporal lobe epilepsy, suicide rates are around 25 times that of the general population.

Schwartz JM and Marsh L. The psychiatric perspectives of epilepsy. *Psychosomatics* 2000; **41**: 31–38.

33. B. Geschwind's syndrome is an eponymous syndrome of interictal behaviour/personality disorder which has been described in temporal lobe epilepsy (TLE). Clinical features of this syndrome include preoccupation with philosophical and religious concerns, anger, excessive emotionality, viscosity (noted especially in speech), circumstantiality, altered sexuality, and hypergraphia. Recent reviews state that personality traits, rather than a personality disorder *per se*, seems more likely in these disorders and they tend to resemble the cluster C category of disorders in DSM-IV.

Marcangelo MJ and Ovsiew F. Psychiatric aspects of epilepsy. *Psychiatric Clinics of North America* 2007; **30**: 781–802.
Swinkelsa WAM, Kuyka J, Dyckb R, and Spinhoven P. Psychiatric comorbidity in epilepsy. *Epilepsy and Behavior* 2005; **7**: 37–50.

34. E.   Psychogenic non-epileptic seizures were previously referred to as 'pseudoseizures'. They are seizure-like behavioural events that occur in the absence of abnormal electrical discharge in the brain. The gold standard for diagnosis is video-EEG monitoring. People who present with non-epileptic seizures commonly have comorbid epilepsy. Nearly 30 to 50% of patients who have non-epileptic seizures have epilepsy and 20 to 60% of patients who have epilepsy have non-epileptic seizures. The average age of onset is between 20 and 30 years and it is three times more common in women than men. Prevalence rates of a history of sexual abuse in non-epileptic seizures range from 25 to 75%. An elevated prolactin level (usually two times baseline or three standard deviations above normal) could be due to seizures or any neurological event, such as syncope. Some patients with pseudoseizures may have modest elevations in prolactin levels. A normal prolactin may not always be diagnostic of pseudoseizures, since it is frequently normal in partial seizures and sampling may be mistimed following convulsions.

Marcangelo MJ and Ovsiew F. Psychiatric aspects of epilepsy. *Psychiatric Clinics of North America* 2007; **30**: 781–802.

35. C.   Historically, left anterior stroke has been associated with depression. This has been questioned in more recent times—including a few meta-analyses that did not show such a relationship. The laterality hypothesis of poststroke depression may hold true only in the acute stage of illness of less than 2 months' duration. As time passes, the chance of getting a depressive episode is equal in all kinds of stroke. Major depression occurs in approximately 10–25% of patients. Anxiety occurs without depression in up to 10%. Apathy occurs in 20% of patients. Anosognosia with denial of illness is present in 25–45% of patients, particularly those with right posterior lesions. Catastrophic reactions appear in approximately 20% and emotional lability is present in 20%. The mean duration of major depression appears to be about 9 months, but can be chronic, lasting for years in hospitalized patients.

Chemerinski E and Robinson GR. The neuropsychiatry of stroke. *Psychosomatics* 2000; **41**: 5–14.

36. C.   Goldstein instigated the term 'catastrophic reaction' to describe a cluster of symptoms characterized by aggressive outbursts in patients with brain injury. It was ascribed to the inability of the person to cope with the physical/cognitive deficit. An important study with respect to catastrophic reaction was conducted by Starkstein *et al.* in 1993. The major findings of this study are as follows. Catastrophic reaction occurs in around 20% of stroke patients. It is associated with a personal and family history of psychiatric illness. It is also significantly associated with the presence of poststroke depression. It is more common in anterior subcortical lesions and lesions involving the basal ganglia. The reaction is not merely a frustration reaction to the presence of aphasia or cognitive deficits; it could be present as a symptom on its own or as a behavioural symptom in a subgroup of depressed patients with anterior subcortical damage.

Starkstein SE, Fedoroff JP, Price TR et al. Catastrophic reaction after cerebrovascular lesions: frequency, correlates, and validation of a scale. *Journal of Neuropsychiatry and Clinical Neuroscience* 1993; **5**: 189–194.

37. B.   On the basis of the fact that not all patients with a left anterior or a right posterior lesion develop depression, other premorbid factors were studied by Starkstein *et al.* Along with the presence of family history of affective disorders in those who developed poststroke depression, they also found that there was no significant relationship between the presence of depression and demographic variables such as age, sex, education, socioeconomic status, etc. Presence of premorbid cortical atrophy was found to be a risk factor for depression. Similarly, cortical atrophy also predicts mania.

Starkstein SE, Robinson RG, and Price TR. Comparison of patients with and without poststroke major depression matched for size and location of lesion. *Archives of General Psychiatry* 1983; **45**: 247–252.

38. B. The middle cerebral artery supplies most of the cortical grey matter, including the parietal cortex. The inferior parietal lobe includes the upper part of the optic radiation which carries fibres from upper half of the retina and hence lesions of this area produce inferior quadrantanopia. Parietal lobe damage also explains the hemineglect, mild hemiparesis, and dressing apraxia. Carotid artery syndrome usually presents with amaurosis fugax, the feature distinguishing it from the middle cerebral artery syndrome. Amaurosis fugax is transient, painless monocular blindness, usually due to emboli either from the large arteries or the heart itself. Occlusions of the coronaries usually occur at the bifurcation of the common carotid.

Kasper DL *et al.*, eds. *Harrison's Principles of Internal Medicine*, 16th edn. McGraw-Hill, 2005, p. 2381.

39. D. Stage 4 NREM sleep is characterized by more than 50% delta activity. When the delta activity ranges from 20 to 50%, the person is in stage 3 NREM sleep. K complexes and sleep spindles along with delta waves of less than 20% is noted in stage 2. Stage 2 is also the longest sleep stage through the night, comprising almost 50% of adult sleep. Stage 1 is characterized by gradual slowing of the alpha wave (less than 50% alpha activity). This is the sleep onset. Stage W (wakefulness) is characterized by predominantly alpha waves posteriorly with low voltage mixed frequency beta waves anteriorly. REM sleep constitutes around 20–25%. Normally, much less time is spent in stage W and stage 1.

Hales RE and Yudofsky SC, eds. *The American Psychiatric Publishing Textbook of Neuropsychiatry and Clinical Neurosciences*, 4th edn. American Psychiatric Press, 2002, p. 698.

40. A. Characteristics of REM sleep include variable heart and breathing rate, high oxygen consumption and cerebral blood flow, penile erections (morning erections due to high levels of REMs), increased vaginal blood flow and uterine activity, absent electrodermal activity, poikilothermic state, and dream-like mental activity. In contrast, NREM sleep is characterized by regular, slow heart and breathing rate, low cerebral blood flow and O_2 consumption, absent penile blood flow, and thought-like mental activity. Muscular tone is maintained in NREM sleep and atonia is seen in REM.

Hales RE and Yudofsky SC, eds. *The American Psychiatric Publishing Textbook of Neuropsychiatry and Clinical Neurosciences*, 4th edn. American Psychiatric Press, 2002, p. 699.

41. A. Sleep terrors occur in slow-wave sleep (stage 3 and 4) unlike nightmares which occur in REM sleep. Sleep terrors are characterized by a sudden arousal with intense fearfulness, often associated with a sharp scream. The subject may sit up in bed, may vocalize unintelligibly, and waking the individual leads to confusion. There is amnesia for the episode and unlike nightmares it is very rarely associated with vividly recalled dreams and images. A familial pattern has been reported. In children, night terrors may be transient but in adults they may be associated with other psychopathology.

Hales RE and Yudofsky SC, eds. *The American Psychiatric Publishing Textbook of Neuropsychiatry and Clinical Neurosciences*, 4th edn. American Psychiatric Press, 2002, p. 717.

42. D. This patient is likely to have narcolepsy. Narcolepsy is a disorder of unknown aetiology. It consists of the tetrad of excessive day time sleepiness, cataplexy, sleep paralysis, and hypnagogic hallucinations. Polysomnography typically shows sleep-onset REM stage. Cataplexy refers to sudden loss of muscular tone, often seen in association with emotional reactions in those with narcolepsy. An abnormality in the hypocretin neurones in the lateral hypothalamus has been noted in those with narcolepsy. Hypocretin (orexin) is a highly excitatory peptide hormone secreted from the hypothalamus. This is necessary to maintain wakefulness and it also increases appetite. Narcolepsy, especially cataplexy, is considered to be a hypocretin deficiency syndrome. SSRIs and TCAs remain the treatment of choice currently. Modafinil is also being tried as a treatment.

Siegel JM, Moore R, Thannickal T, and Nienhuis R. A brief history of hypocretin/orexin and narcolepsy. *Neuropsychopharmacology* 2001; **25**: S14–S20.

43. D. Dementia is estimated to occur in 27% of patients with Parkinson's disease (PD). Dementia has been associated with older age, greater PD severity, hallucinations, longer duration of PD, greater disability, and male gender. Causes of dementia in PD include Lewy body pathology, dopamine depletion, coexisting AD, and other conditions. Reduced fluorodopa uptake in the frontal cortex and caudate nucleus, and in mesolimbic pathways are predictors of cognitive impairment. Temporoparietal cortical hypometabolism also predicts cognitive impairment. Donepezil has been found to be useful in two separate double-blind trials in patients with PD.

Lauterbach CE. The neuropsychiatry of Parkinson's disease and related disorders. *Psychiatric Clinics of North America* 2004; **27**: 801–825.

44. C. Progressive supranuclear palsy is considered as a Parkinson plus syndrome. It is distinguished from Parkinson's disease by the presence of early broad-based and stiff gait disorder (axial greater than limb rigidity in extension) with backward falls, and supranuclear gaze palsy with slow vertical saccades and difficulty looking down (and hence the falls). Falls are very common in these patients and are an important cause of morbidity. Patients are prone to develop various psychiatric complications, including cognitive dysfunction and mood disorders. Cholinesterase inhibitors have not been particularly useful in treating patients with progressive supranuclear palsy associated dementia. Other Parkinson plus syndromes include multisystem atrophy (called Shy–Drager syndrome when associated with autonomic failure), olivopontocerebellar atrophy, and corticobasal degeneration.

Lauterbach CE. The neuropsychiatry of Parkinson's disease and related disorders. *Psychiatric Clinics of North America* 2004; **27**: 801–825.

45. C. In this case the origin of emboli must be at the internal carotid artery. The ophthalmic artery, a branch of the internal carotid artery, is blocked transiently, producing the symptoms described in the question. This is called as amaurosis fugax which translates to 'fleeting darkness'. It is related to transient but sudden monocular visual loss as a result of decreased retinal circulation. It is a type of transient ischaemic attack and could be a harbinger of a cerebrovascular accident. Compromise of posterior circulation usually leads to cortical blindness, often with macular sparing.

Darby D and Walsh K. *Neuropsychology: A Clinical Approach*, 5th edn. Elsevier, 2005, p. 84.

46. A. The given history is consistent with dissociative fugue. Fugue states are associated with stressful life events wherein total amnesia for the recent past can be seen. More often the amnesia related to dissociation is circumscribed to events of personal importance. During the fugue, the patient may retain normal functional activities and may even learn new verbal and non-verbal materials. Following recovery from the fugue, one may not remember the activities carried out during the fugue state.

Darby D and Walsh K. *Neuropsychology: A Clinical Approach*, 5th edn. Elsevier, 2005, p. 101.

47. C. This is an example of utilization behaviour. A patient with utilization behaviour will be forced to 'utilize' objects presented to him despite the absence of obvious need for such usage. An extreme form of this is seen in 'environmental dependence syndrome'—the patient becomes compelled to make use of all that is seen in his immediate environment resulting in an array of serial complex behaviour. Klüver–Bucy syndrome occurs in the context of bilateral temporal lobe damage. It is associated with hyperorality, inappropriate sexuality, and increased exploratory behaviour (hypermetamorphosis). Alien hand syndrome refers to loss of control of limb movements resulting in 'automatic' coordinated hand movements. The patient is usually aware of this and may try to exercise control using the other hand. Balint's syndrome is characterized by oculomotor apraxia, optic ataxia, and simultanagnosia.

Darby D and Walsh K. *Neuropsychology: A Clinical Approach*, 5th edn. Elsevier, 2005, p. 132.

48. A. Utilization behaviour is seen in patients with frontal lobe damage. Dominant parietal lobe lesions result in apraxia, right–left confusion, acalculia, and finger agnosia. Balint's syndrome occurs in bilateral parieto-occipital damage.

Ropper AH and Brown RH, eds. *Adam and Victor's Principles of Neurology*, 8th edn. McGraw-Hill, 2005, p. 391.

49. D. Temporal lobe is the most common site of origin of complex partial seizures; in very few cases parietal focus has been demonstrated. When accompanied by hallucinations, intense emotional reactions may be seen during the seizure. Fear is the most common emotion noted. Curiously, patients are often aware of the unreal nature of their hallucinatory experiences, but this awareness is not specific to complex seizures. Pathology of familiarity characterized by *déjà vu* and *jamais vu* are commonly reported in temporal lobe epilepsy.

Ropper AH and Brown RH, eds. *Adam and Victor's Principles of Neurology*, 8th edn. McGraw-Hill, 2005, p. 277.

50. B. Progressive fluent aphasia early in the course of a dementing illness is a feature of semantic dementia. Semantic dementia is a type of frontotemporal degenerative disorder. The pathological finding is predominantly frontotemporal degeneration with ubiquitin inclusions. Motor neurone disease type inclusions may also be noted. Semantic memory refers to representation of meanings, understanding concepts, and knowledge unrelated to temporal events (cf. episodic memory). Focal cortical deficits, especially progressive aphasia, can be presenting features of Alzheimer's disease but this is uncommon.

Alladi J, Xuereb T, Bak P *et al.* Focal cortical presentations of Alzheimer's disease. *Brain* 2007; **130**: 2636–2645.

51. A. The National Adult Reading Test (NART) has been widely used as a measure of premorbid IQ. The usefulness of NART as a measure of premorbid IQ is based on two assumptions:
1. Reading ability is relatively independent of brain damage.
2. Ability to read irregular words from a list is a strong predictor of intelligence in the normal population.

Hence in those with brain damage, irrespective of the diagnosis, NART can be used to estimate the most probable IQ level before becoming ill. However, the notion that the NART score is relatively independent of brain damage has come under scrutiny of late. Studies in Alzheimer's dementia and Korsakoff's syndrome have indicated deterioration in reading ability, leading to an underestimated premorbid IQ.

Bright P, Jaldow E, and Kopelman MD. The National Adult Reading Test as a measure of premorbid intelligence: A comparison with estimates derived from demographic variables. *Journal of the International Neuropsychological Society* 2002; **8**: 847–854.

52. D. This history is consistent with transient global amnesia (TGA). Sudden-onset amnesia with inability to form new memories of current events and a variable degree of retrograde amnesia is seen. The entire episode lasts for hours to days and on recovery the extent of retrograde amnesia shrinks and almost intact memory for events that happened before the episode is restored, but a dense amnesia persists for the events during the episode (24 hours in this case) even after full recovery. During the episode itself, the procedural memory, visuospatial functions, and problem-solving ability are intact; the patients may even be able to drive during the episode.

Ropper AH and Brown RH, eds. *Adam and Victor's Principles of Neurology*, 8th edn. McGraw-Hill, 2005, p. 379.

53. C. TGA is thought to be vascular in origin. Posterior cerebral circulation (vertebrobasilar insufficiency) is implicated, which supplies significant part of hippocampal and other medial temporal regions. Migrainous or epileptic aetiology has not been entirely disproved. Obstruction to cortical sinuses may be related to idiopathic intracranial hypertension in some cases. The middle meningeal artery may be injured in skull fractures, often becoming a source of extradural haematoma.

Ropper AH and Brown RH, eds. *Adam and Victor's Principles of Neurology*, 8th edn. McGraw-Hill, 2005, p. 379.

54. C. The anterior spinothalamic tract is supplied by the anterior spinal artery. The spinothalamic tract carries pain and temperature sensations. Posterior tracts such as dorsal columns of gracilis and cuneatus carry joint sense, light touch, proprioception, and vibration sensations. Infarction of the spinal cord usually involves the territory of the anterior spinal artery—the ventral two-thirds of the spinal cord.

Ropper AH and Brown RH, eds. *Adam and Victor's Principles of Neurology*, 8th edn. McGraw-Hill, 2005, p. 1069.

55. A. The cerebellum has an external cortical grey matter and the deep cerebellar nuclei. There are four deep nuclei: dentate, globose, emboli-form, and fastigial nuclei. Mossy fibres and climbing fibres provide the major input into the cerebellum. Substantia nigra and subthalamic nucleus are part of basal ganglia. Red nucleus is an upper brainstem nucleus seen at the level of tegmentum. Similar to substantia nigra, red nucleus also contains iron pigments. It is involved in motor coordination.

Ropper AH and Brown RH, eds. *Adam and Victor's Principles of Neurology*, 8th edn. McGraw-Hill, 2005, p. 73.

56. C. Pseudobulbar palsy is also known as spastic bulbar palsy. It usually results from bilateral frontal damage. This may be due to vascular, demyelinating, or motor neurone disease (amyotrophic lateral sclerosis). Diffuse brainstem damage (bulb) will produce lesions in the cranial nerve nuclei, causing bulbar palsy. Pseudobulbar palsy is an upper motor neurone type of lesion. Bulbar palsy produces lower motor neurone damage. Hence increased tone (producing spastic tongue), exaggerated tendon reflexes (brisk jaw jerk), and lack of fasciculations are notable. Diffuse frontal damage may produce frontal release signs. Poliomyelitis, diptheria, and Guillain–Barré syndrome are known causes. The most common cause of progressive bulbar palsy is motor neurone disease.

Ropper AH and Brown RH, eds. *Adam and Victor's Principles of Neurology*, 8th edn. McGraw-Hill, 2005, p. 1187 and 426.

57. B.   Lesions of the subthalamic nucleus are associated with hemiballismus. Lesions of the caudate nucleus are associated with chorea. Disturbances in the GABA system of caudate nucleus are noted in Huntington's disease. Similarly, damage to the caudate nucleus is implicated in Sydenham's chorea seen in streptococcal infection. Parkinsonian movement disturbances, especially bradykinesia, are associated with damage to the substantia nigra.

Ropper AH and Brown RH, eds. *Adam and Victor's Principles of Neurology*, 8th edn. McGraw-Hill, 2005, p. 61.

58. C.   Set shifting is an executive function. In the Wisconsin Card Sorting Test, abstract reasoning and flexibility in problem solving are tested. In this test, cards of different colour, form, and number are available. Patients are asked to sort the cards into groups according to varying categories (colour only, form only, or number only) as requested by the examiner. This measures the capacity for abstract thinking and set-shifting ability (cognitive flexibility). Tower of London is a problem-solving test; it involves frontal and basal ganglia function but does not directly test set-shifting ability. Rey Osterrieth figure is a test of visual memory wherein a complex geometric figure is given to be copied, followed by immediate reproduction from memory and reproduction after a delay.

Sadock BJ and Sadock VA. *Kaplan and Sadock's Synopsis of Psychiatry: Behavioral Sciences/Clinical Psychiatry*, 10th edn. Lippincott Williams and Wilkins, 2007, p. 184.

59. C.   Anomic (or nominal) aphasia presents with inability to name objects and body parts. Patients have fluent speech, intact repetition, intact comprehension, reading, and writing. Nominal aphasia often presents together with, or may follow, recovery from other forms of aphasia. Nominal aphasia is not very useful for lesion localization. It is also noted in early Alzheimer's disease.

Ropper AH and Brown RH, eds. *Adam and Victor's Principles of Neurology*, 8th edn. McGraw-Hill, 2005, p. 422.

60. D.   The blood supply to the rostral third of the hippocampus comes from the anterior choroidal artery, which is a direct branch of the internal carotid artery. It does not take part in the circle of Willis anastamosis. The occipital two-thirds are supplied by hippocampal branches, the posteromedial choroidal artery, and the inferior temporal branches of the posterior cerebral artery.

Lüdemann W, Schneekloth C, Samii M, and Hussein S. Arterial supply of the temporo-medial region of the brain significance for preoperative vascular occlusion testing. *Surgical and Radiologic Anatomy* 2001; **23**: 39–43.

61. D.   Early in the Alzheimer's disease neuronal loss is most pronounced in layer II of the entorhinal cortex of the hippocampus. The parahippocampal gyri and subiculum are also affected. This extends to anterior nuclei of the thalamus, septal nuclei, amygdala, and monoaminergic systems of the brainstem are also depleted. The cholinergic neurones of the nucleus basalis of Meynert are also reduced. In cerebral cortex, most pronounced loss occurs with respect to pyramidal neurones and astrocytic proliferation follows as a compensatory or reparative process, most prominently in layers III and V.

Ropper AH and Brown RH, eds. *Adam and Victor's Principles of Neurology*, 8th edn. McGraw-Hill, 2005, p. 901.

62. A. Excessive stimulation of glutamate receptors leads to an increase in intraneuronal calcium and nitric oxide. Calcium activates proteases that could destroy the neurone from within. Memantine is an NMDA antagonist used in the treatment of Alzheimer's disease, based on the excitotoxicity hypothesis. This mechanism may be applicable for Parkinson's disease too. In Huntington's disease, an expansion of the polyglutamine region of huntingtin takes place due to the disease-causing mutation. Hence the mutant huntingtin protein accumulates in the nuclei of neurones, preferentially in striatum and cortex. These aggregates may be directly toxic to some extent, but predominant striatal loss, as opposed to cortical loss, may be due to glutamate-mediated excitotoxicity. Huntingtin accumulation may render cells unusually sensitive to glutamate-mediated damage.

Ropper AH and Brown RH, eds. *Adam and Victor's Principles of Neurology*, 8th edn. McGraw-Hill, 2005, p. 912.

63. D. Posterior inferior cerebellar artery occlusion leads to Wallenberg's syndrome. The resulting signs and symptoms are attributed to infarction of a wedge of lateral medulla that contains vestibular nuclei, descending sympathetic tract, spoinothalamic system (carrying pain and temperature from contralateral side of body), descending fifth nerve tract and nucleus, and ninth and tenth nerve fibres of same side. This leads to ipsilateral Horner's syndrome (miopsis, anhidrosis, and ptosis due to sympathetic damage), ipsilateral loss of face sensation (fifth nerve damage), dysphagia, hoarseness, loss of gag reflex (ninth/tenth nerve damage), and contralateral loss of pain and temperature over half of the body.

Ropper AH and Brown RH, eds. *Adam and Victor's Principles of Neurology*, 8th edn. McGraw-Hill, 2005, p. 679.

64. A. The age of the patient, the triad of memory difficulties, loss of balance, and urinary incontinence, and the neuroimaging findings suggest normal-pressure hydrocephalus (NPH). NPH is not a hydrocephalus in the true sense—there is no increase in intracranial pressure when lumbar puncture is carried out. Following certain meningeal insults, secondary to subarachnoid haemorrhage, head trauma, or resolved meningitis, an increase in intracranial pressure may develop but reach a stable stage where formation of CSF diminishes and equilibrates with absorption, which increases proportionate to the pressure. Once this equilibrium is reached there must be a gradual fall in pressure, although at a high normal level. In some patients, this high normal intracranial pressure of 150 to 200 mm H_2O leads to manifestation of NPH.

Ropper AH and Brown RH, eds. *Adam and Victor's Principles of Neurology*, 8th edn. McGraw-Hill, 2005, p. 535.

65. B. The presence of low heart rate, muscle tone, and blood pressure is suggestive of NREM sleep. At this stage of sleep if a person is awakened, he will be confused. He may not recollect the instance of awakening in the morning. A normal adult spends nearly 75% of sleep in various NREM stages, while the remaining 25% is REM sleep. Penile erection, high cerebral blood flow, and vividly recalled dreams are features of REM stage.

Ropper AH and Brown RH, eds. *Adam and Victor's Principles of Neurology*, 8th edn. McGraw-Hill, 2005, p. 335.

66. B. Alpha, beta, delta, and theta are four important wavelets in EEG when awake. Alpha waves are predominant, especially posteriorly when the eyes are closed; they occur at a frequency of 8 to 13 Hz. Beta waves are sometimes seen in normal EEG over central, anterior regions; they occur at a frequency higher than 13 Hz. Theta activity is seen infrequently when awake but often when a subject is drowsy or sleeping. Excessive theta when awake is abnormal. Delta waves (frequency less than 3.5 Hz) are normally seen only in deep sleep and are pathological if noted in adult waking EEG. With ageing, slow waves become more common in EEG.

Sadock BJ and Sadock VA. *Kaplan and Sadock's Synopsis of Psychiatry: Behavioral Sciences/Clinical Psychiatry*, 10th edn. Lippincott Williams and Wilkins, 2007, p. 118.

67. A. Huntington's disease is characterized by diffuse flattening or loss of alpha waves in EEG. In a study conducted in a group of 95 patients with Huntington's chorea, 31 showed little activity of any kind (flat trace EEG) and in particular no alpha rhythm above 10 µV in amplitude was seen. There was a statistically significant association between cortical atrophy, especially the frontal lobe, and a 'low voltage' EEG in the same study. Such low-voltage records, though not specific for Huntington's chorea, are rare in other neurological disorders.

Scott DF, Heathfield KWG, Toone B, and Margerison JH. The EEG in Huntington's chorea: a clinical and neuropathological study. *Journal of Neurology, Neurosurgery and Psychiatry* 1972; **35**: 97–102.

68. E. Two types of cannabinoid receptors, central (CB1) and peripheral (CB2), have been identified. Both receptors bind to exogenously administered tetrahydrocannabinol (THC), present in marijuana. Anandamide (from the Sanskrit word 'ananda' for bliss) is chemically *N*-arachidonoylethanolamine (arachidonic acid and ethanolamine derivative). It is a weak endogenous cannabinoid ligand. 2-arachnidonylglycerol is a strong endogenous ligand for the cannabinoid receptor. Endogenous cannabinoids exhibit intraocular pressure-lowering effects. They also decrease motor activity level and relieve pain. Anandamides are demonstrated in the thalamus, with a putative role in pain-related neurotransmission.

Sadock BJ and Sadock VA. *Kaplan and Sadock's Synopsis of Psychiatry: Behavioral Sciences/Clinical Psychiatry*, 10th edn. Lippincott Williams and Wilkins, 2007, p. 110.

69. D. Bitemporal hemianopia is secondary to chiasmatic lesions. Pituitary tumours characteristically cause bitemporal hemianopia. Craniopharyngioma is a benign epithelioid tumour arising from remnants of Rathke's pouch at the junction of the infundibular stem and pituitary. It lies above the sella turcica and so exerts pressure effects on the optic chiasm leading to bitemporal hemianopia. Tunnel vision is a result of extensive peripheral field defects. Quadrantanopias usually result from damage to the optic radiation beyond the chiasma. Parietal lesions result in inferior, while temporal lesions result in superior, quadrantanopia.

Ropper AH and Brown RH, eds. *Adam and Victor's Principles of Neurology*, 8th edn. McGraw-Hill, 2005, p. 574.

70. C. Priapism is defined as a persistent penile erection greater than 4 hours in duration, which is unrelated to sexual stimulation or desire. Roughly 40 to 50% of patients who develop priapism become impotent, even after surgical treatment. Drug-induced priapism accounts for 15–40% of all cases. Psychotropics associated with priapism include trazodone, phenothiazines, butyrophenones, risperidone, and clozapine. Priapism results from decreased venous outflow from the corpora cavernosa of the penis. This can be caused by obstruction of the venous system, for example by blood dyscrasias such as sickle cell anaemia or by blocking the sympathetically mediated (α_1 receptor) detumescence. Hence the ability of a drug to block α_1 receptors correlates with its risk of priapism. This is especially true if the antiadrenergic effect is unopposed by an equally strong anticholinergic effect. Sympathetic tone is related to detumescence while parasympathetic tone is related to erection. For drugs with combined antiadrenergic and anticholinergic activity, when antiadrenergic activity negates detumescence, the anticholinergic activity will negate erection and so priapism will be rare.

Heckers S, Anick D, Boverman JF, and Stern TA. Priapism following olanzapine administration in a patient with multiple sclerosis. *Psychosomatics* 1998; **39**: 288–290.

71. B. Metacognition refers to one's knowledge concerning one's own cognitive processes and products of such processes. Metacognition is predominantly a function of prefrontal cortex. Prefrontal damage leads to overestimation of abilities, lack of awareness of deficits, and inability to use feedback to change behaviour.

Fernandez-Duque D, Baird J, and Posner MI. Executive attention and metacognitive regulation. *Consciousness and Cognition* 2000; **9**: 288–307.

72. A. 'N back' test is a popular experimental paradigms for functional neuroimaging studies of working memory. In this test subjects are asked to monitor a series of verbal or non-verbal stimuli and to indicate when the currently presented stimulus is the same as the one presented n trials previously. Using quantitative meta-analysis technique of normative functional imaging studies, a broadly consistent activation of frontal and parietal cortical regions by various versions of the n-back working memory paradigm has been demonstrated.

Owen AM, McMillan KM, Laird AR, and Bullmore E. N-back working memory paradigm: a meta-analysis of normative functional neuroimaging studies. *Human Brain Mapping* 2005; **25**: 46–59.

73. B. MPTP occurred as an impurity when illicit synthesis of opioids was attempted by a chemistry graduate student. He developed acute parkinsonian disease. Following detailed investigations, animal models of Parkinson's disease have been developed using MPTP as a neurotoxin. VMA is a metabolite of epinephrine; 5HIAA is a metabolite of serotonin. MDMA is the chemical name for ecstasy. Ketamine is a dissociative anaesthetic that stimulates sigma receptors in brain. It is being increasingly used as a street drug.

Johnstone EC *et al.*, eds. *Companion to Psychiatric Studies*, 7th edn. Churchill Livingstone, 2004, p. 10.

74. D. Human neocortex consists of a six-layered laminar structure. This cytoarchitectural division has been largely adapted from Brodmann's pioneering work. These six layers are numbered from the top, that is the pial surface to the underlying white matter. In order, these are:
1. Molecular (or plexiform)
2. External granular layer
3. External pyramidal
4. Internal granular
5. Internal pyramidal (or ganglionic)
6. Multiform (or fusiform) layer.
The layers vary mostly in the size and density of pyramidal and stellate cells.

Johnstone EC *et al.*, eds. *Companion to Psychiatric Studies*, 7th edn. Churchill Livingstone, 2004, p. 11.

75. E. Lateral geniculate nucleus is the junction where axons of retinal ganglion cells terminate after passing through uninterrupted via the optic nerve, optic chiasm, and optic tract. The medial geniculate body is involved in auditory processing.

Johnstone EC *et al.*, eds. *Companion to Psychiatric Studies*, 7th edn. Churchill Livingstone, 2004, p. 12.

76. D. Granule cells are the only excitatory neurones in the cerebellum. The cerebellar cortex is a three-layered structure with the outermost layer containing two types of inhibitory neurones, the stellate cells and basket cells. The middle layer has cell bodies of Purkinje cells (main output) which are GABA-mediated and so are inhibitory in function. The innermost layer contains granule cells, which are excitatory, and Golgi cells, which are inhibitory.

Johnstone EC *et al.*, eds. *Companion to Psychiatric Studies*, 7th edn. Churchill Livingstone, 2004, p. 17.

77. A. Working memory can be tested using digit span tasks. Using digit repetition forward, a patient's working memory capacity can be tested. Usually, a list of numbers (in no specific pattern) is read aloud by the examiner and the patient is asked to repeat it immediately in same order (forward span) or reverse order (backward span). Gradually, the length of the numeric string is increased. Consistent error at a particular length is an indication for test termination. The normal forward digit span is 7±2 for most adults. Backward span is more difficult and averages around 5±2.

Conklin HM, Curtis CE, Katsanis J, and Iacono WG. Verbal working memory impairment in schizophrenia patients and their first-degree relatives: evidence from the Digit Span Task. *American Journal of Psychiatry* 2000; **157**: 275–277.

78. C. Sensory ataxia is due to posterior column disease, resulting from spinal cord lesions. In this condition, loss of joint position sense and loss of tendon reflexes are seen. In cerebellar ataxia, associated cerebellar signs such as dysarthria or nystagmus may be present. The corrective effects of vision on balance and posture are seen in sensory ataxia. This is elicited by Romberg's test wherein swaying, which is almost absent when eyes are open and feet together, becomes prominent on eye closure. In cerebellar ataxia, the patient may sway even with eyes open, which worsens on eye closure.

Ropper AH and Brown RH, eds. *Adam and Victor's Principles of Neurology*, 8th edn. McGraw-Hill, 2005, p. 79.

79. C. Long-term potentiation (LTP) is conceptualized as a more or less permanent increase in synaptic efficacy following high-frequency activity across the synapse. Glutamate via NMDA receptor activation influences LTP. This may underlie changes in synaptic plasticity observed in learning- and memory-related processes. LTP is proposed to be the cellular biological correlate of long-term memory.

Johnstone EC *et al.*, eds. *Companion to Psychiatric Studies*, 7th edn. Churchill Livingstone, 2004, p. 28.

80. B. Most neurones from the ventral tegmental area of midbrain ascend in the medial forebrain bundle and the nigrostriatal pathway. These neurones are rich in dopamine. The dopamine neurones of the ventral tegmental area (VTA) are thought to play a central role in reward, motivation, and drug addiction. Nucleus basalis of Meynert is a major cholinergic site. Dorsal raphe nucleus is predominantly a serotonergic site. Locus coeruleus contains noradrenergic neurones.

Johnstone EC *et al.*, eds. *Companion to Psychiatric Studies*, 7th edn. Churchill Livingstone, 2004, p. 31.

81. A. Nucleus basalis of Meynert contains a majority of cholinergic neurones. Apart from hippocampal (entorhinal cortex) neuronal loss, selective loss of neurones in the nucleus basalis has led to the pursuit of cholinergic theories of memory impairment in dementia. Currently available pharmacological interventions largely target cholinergic deficiency in Alzheimer's disease.

Wilcock GK, Esiri MM, Bowen DM, and Smiths CCT. The nucleus basalis in Alzheimer's disease: cell counts and cortical biochemistry. *Neuropathology and Applied Neurobiology* 1982; **9**: 175–179.

82. C. SM, a patient with rare bilateral amygdala damage, was initially reported to lack the ability to recognize fear from facial expressions. Since the report of her case, a number of lesion and functional imaging studies have demonstrated the role of the amygdala in fear processing. It is possible that the amygdala mediates spontaneous fixations on the eyes when viewing expressions of faces. Lack of such fixation may lead to failure of spontaneous processing of fearful emotions.

Adolphs R, Gosselin F, Buchanan TW *et al*. A mechanism for impaired fear recognition after amygdala damage. *Nature* 2005; **433**: 68–72.

83. A. Pyridoxine (vitamin B$_6$) when phosphorylated to pyridoxal phosphate acts as a coenzyme in the conversion of glutamic acid to GABA, mediated by the rate-limiting enzyme glutamate decarboxylase. The pivotal role of this chemical interaction is evident from pyridoxine-dependent seizures, which can occur in relation to mutations of chromosome 5q31. Dysfunction of this enzyme leads to glutamate accumulation and excitatory damage via NMDA receptors.

Tan H, Kardaşlu F, Büyükavci M, and Karakelleoğlu C. Pyridoxine-dependent seizures and microcephaly. *Paediatric Neurology* 2004; **31**: 211–213.

84. C. The circumventricular organs are midline structures around the third and fourth ventricles. Pineal gland, median eminence, neurohypophysis, subfornical organ, area postrema, subcommissural organ, organum vasculosum of the lamina terminalis, and the choroid plexus are considered as circumventricular organs. These structures lack the blood–brain barrier seen in other regions of brain. These areas enable the brain's direct response to chemical challenges in blood.

Johnstone EC *et al*., eds. *Companion to Psychiatric Studies*, 7th edn. Churchill Livingstone, 2004, p. 38.

85. C. A neuromodulator is a substance that enhances or diminishes the effect of neurotransmitters but does not usually result in neuronal conduction changes on its own. Substance P, enkephalin, cholecystokinin, somatostatin, and neuropeptide Y are examples of neuromodulators. Neurotrophin is a substance produced to influence neuronal growth. Neurohormones are substances released by neurones into the blood stream to influence effector organs at distant sites, for example corticotrophin-releasing hormone.

Johnstone EC *et al*., eds. *Companion to Psychiatric Studies*, 7th edn. Churchill Livingstone, 2004, p. 41.

86. D. Norepinephrine acts as physiological antagonist for acetylcholine. Physiological antagonism is defined as the process wherein two chemical molecules that act through two different receptor systems result in opposing actions in the body that tend to negate each other's physiological effect. Insulin and glucagon can be considered as physiological antagonists, to some extent.

Johnstone EC *et al*., eds. *Companion to Psychiatric Studies*, 7th edn. Churchill Livingstone, 2004, p. 42.

87. E.   Muscarinic receptors act via the G protein-coupled second messenger system. Nicotinic cholinergic receptors operate via ligand gated channels that are permeable to Na^+, K^+ and sometimes Ca^{2+}. $GABA_A$ receptors are also ligand-gated ion channels that allow Cl^- ions to pass through, resulting in inhibitory activity. Glycine receptors are strychnine-sensitive ligand-gated ion channels with inhibitory activity. Metabotropic receptors aside, most glutamate receptors (NMDA, AMPA, and kainate) are ionotropic and allow Ca^{2+} transit (NMDA, AMPA) or Na^+, K^+ transit (kainate) via ligand-gated channels.

Johnstone EC *et al.*, eds. *Companion to Psychiatric Studies*, 7th edn. Churchill Livingstone, 2004, p. 43.

88. D. ^{11}C raclopride is used to identify postsynaptic dopamine receptors (D2/D3). Raclopride is related to the antipsychotic sulpride and amisulpride (substituted benzamide); hence it acts as a D2/D3 inhibitor.

Johnstone EC *et al.*, eds. *Companion to Psychiatric Studies*, 7th edn. Churchill Livingstone, 2004, p. 79.

89. D.   Adipose tissues are the major source of leptin. The amount of leptin in plasma is directly proportional to degree of adiposity in one's body. Leptin enters the brain, by an unknown mechanism, to reduce appetite via a central mechanism. In obesity, a certain degree of leptin resistance exists, leading to high circulating levels of leptin.

Mantzoros CS. Leptin and the hypothalamus: neuroendocrine regulation of food intake. *Molecular Psychiatry* 1999; **4**: 8–12.

90. E.   Thyroid hormone acts in a similar manner to steroid hormone. Receptors for these hormones are not present in the cell membrane but, upon cellular entry, they bind to nuclear receptors to directly affect cellular processes. These nuclear receptors act as hormone-activated transcription factors that modulate gene expression.

Brent GA. Mechanisms of disease: the molecular basis of thyroid hormone action. *New England Journal of Medicine* 1994; **331**: 847–853.

91. B.   The patient described in the question is most likely to have a diagnosis of Alzheimer's dementia. Diffuse and neuritic plaques with amyloid deposits in cortex and hippocampus are highly suggestive of Alzheimer's disease. Ballooning of cells with intraneuronal accumulations suggests Pick's disease. Diffuse amyloid deposition restricted to blood vessels is seen in amyloid angiopathy. Eosinophilic rod-shaped inclusions of actin filaments are Hirano bodies, seen sometimes in Alzheimer's disease.

Ropper AH and Brown RH, eds. *Adam and Victor's Principles of Neurology*, 8th edn. McGraw-Hill, 2005, p. 899.

92. A. $5-HT_{1B}$ receptors are present as presynaptic autoreceptors. On stimulation, these receptors can decrease further serotonin release. Postsynaptic $5-HT_{1B}$ receptors may have a role in locomotor activity and aggression. $5-HT_{1A}$ receptors are associated with antidepressant activity. $5-HT_{2A}$ receptors are implicated in hallucinogenic properties of LSD-like drugs and blockade is associated with antipsychotic activity. $5-HT_3$ is the only ligand-gated ion channel among serotonin receptors; it is present in gut in large numbers and may mediate emesis.

Sadock BJ and Sadock VA. *Kaplan and Sadock's Synopsis of Psychiatry: Behavioral Sciences/Clinical Psychiatry*, 10th edn. Lippincott Williams and Wilkins, 2007, p. 110.

93. B.   Dopamine exerts its action via one of two families of dopamine receptors. After receptor stimulation, dopamine can either be taken back into the presynaptic neurone and destroyed or repackaged as a neurotransmitter. Among those dopamines that are taken back, some are metabolized by monoamine oxidase (MAO). MAO$_B$ selectively metabolizes dopamine. Catechol-O-methyltransferase (COMT) is localized in the postsynaptic neuronal cytoplasm and is involved in secondary metabolism of dopamine. The primary metabolite of dopamine is homovanillic acid (HVA).

Sadock BJ and Sadock VA. *Kaplan and Sadock's Synopsis of Psychiatry: Behavioral Sciences/Clinical Psychiatry*, 10th edn. Lippincott Williams and Wilkins, 2007, p. 99.

94. B.   In depression, hypercortisolism is seen in a subgroup of patients. This can be demonstrated by the dexamethasone suppression test wherein exogenously administered steroid dexamethasone fails to activate the negative feedback loop to reduce endogenous cortisol. Depressed patients also show blunted TSH response when thyrotrophin-releasing hormone (TRH) is injected. A brisk GH release seen on apomorphine/levodopa challenge is absent in some patients with depression. This suggests dopaminergic dysfunction in a subgroup. Clomipramine challenge in normal subjects leads to increased serotonergic activation and prolactin release. This prolactin response to clomipramine-mediated via serotonin is blunted in depression. Psychotic depression shows more HPA axis disturbance than non-psychotic depression. Melancholic (somatic syndrome) depression increases the chance of finding endocrine disturbances among depressed patients.

Gelder M, López-Ibor J, and Andreasen N. *New Oxford Textbook of Psychiatry*, 1st edn. Oxford University Press, 2003, p. 711–719.

95. D.   P300 is a positive component that occurs 250–500 ms after stimulus onset. Amplitude and latency of P300 is altered in schizophrenia. These changes reflect a trait rather than being related to psychotic state, but these are not specific to schizophrenia; for instance Alzheimer's disease patients show similar deficits. The reduction in amplitude is more pronounced in earlier-onset and paranoid subgroups. P300 is not affected by medication status, disease duration, or severity of psychopathology.

Sadock BJ and Sadock VA. *Kaplan and Sadock's Comprehensive Textbook of Psychiatry*, 8th edn. Lippincott Williams and Wilkins, 2005, p. 200.

96. C.   Fluid intelligence includes non-verbal intellectual functions such as problem solving and reasoning; these are not influenced by one's cultural experience or education. Crystallized intelligence includes acquired knowledge, which is heavily influenced by culture, formal education, and opportunities. Kaufman Adolescent and Adult Intelligence Test measures both 'fluid' and 'crystallized' intelligence. The Wechsler Intelligence Scale for Children and the Wechsler Adult Intelligence Scale measure IQ and are influenced by cultural differences and formal educational attainment. Stanford–Binet Scale is one of the earliest intelligence scales and is influenced by school education. Raven's Progressive Matrix is a measure of ability to form perceptual relations and analogical reason; it is independent of language and formal schooling. It can be used for anyone above age 6.

Raven J. The Raven's Progressive Matrices: change and stability over culture and time. *Cognitive Psychology* 2000; **41**: 1–48.

97. C. Pro-opiomelanocortin (POMC) is a polypeptide precursor protein. It produces many biologically active peptides including the melanocyte-stimulating hormones (MSH), corticotrophin (ACTH), and β-endorphin. MSH and ACTH are collectively known as melanocortins and a family of specific receptors has been described for them. In the CNS, POMC-producing neurones are located in the arcuate nucleus of the hypothalamus and the nucleus tractus solitarius of the brainstem. The CNS POMC system regulates feeding behaviour, sexual behaviour, lactation, the reproductive cycle, and possibly central cardiovascular control.

Millington, GWM. The role of proopiomelanocortin (POMC) neurones in feeding behaviour. *Nutrition and Metabolism* 2007; **4**: 18.

98. B. GABA does not directly mediate working memory. Prefrontal dopamine via D_1 receptors is thought to heavily influence working memory capacity. $GABA_A$ activation has sedative properties. $GABA_A$ activation leads to an increase in seizure threshold via inhibitory activity. $GABA_A$ also plays a role in memory consolidation. GABA agonists prevent formation of long-term memory, though the process of learning itself may not be affected. $GABA_B$ activation mediates central muscle relaxation via spinal cord and brain receptors.

Dash PK, Moore AN, Kobori N, and Runyan JD. Molecular activity underlying working memory. *Learning and Memory* 2007; **14**: 554–563.

99. D. Several neuroanatomical differences between homosexuals and heterosexuals have been reported from human studies. The suprachiasmatic nucleus (SCN) has been noted to be larger and more elongated in homosexual males (and females in general). The third interstitial nucleus of the anterior hypothalamus (INAH-3) was noted to be smaller among homosexuals. Anterior commissure is larger in homosexual men than in heterosexual men. No sexual-orientation differences have been reported in the sexually dimorphic nuclei of the preoptic area in humans.

LeVay S. A difference in hypothalamic structure between heterosexual and homosexual men. *Science* 1991; **253**: 1034–1037.

100. E. Lewy bodies contain ubiquitin (non-specific) and alpha synuclein. Synucleiopathies refer to a set of disorders in which aggregates of synculein accumulation is noted. Lewy bodies are demonstrated pathologically in these disorders, but unlike the Lewy bodies in the substantia nigra seen in Parkinson's disease, cortical Lewy bodies are not surrounded by a distinct halo that enables their identification. Recently, the development of immunostaining for ubiquitin and synuclein have increased the accuracy of visualizing Lewy bodies.

Ropper AH and Brown RH, eds. *Adams and Victor's Principles of Neurology*, 8th edn. McGraw-Hill, 2005, p. 908.

101. E. Wilson's disease is also known as hepatolenticular degeneration. It is an autosomal recessive disorder of copper metabolism. The abnormal gene (*ATP7B*) is located in chromosome 13. Ceruloplasmin is an α_2 globulin that normally carries 90% of the copper present in the plasma. In Wilson's disease, ceruloplasmin fails to bind copper and its excretion by the liver is impaired. The excess copper accumulates first in the liver and then in the brain (especially putamen and pallidus) and other tissues. In the early stages of the disease, proliferation of large protoplasmic astrocytes, such as Opalski cells and Alzheimer cells, occurs. Deposition of copper in Descemet's membrane in the cornea leads to the appearance of the golden-brown 'Kayser–Fleischer' (KF) ring. The main neurological abnormalities are rigidity, dystonia, chorea, athetosis, dysarthria, and tremor. It is considered that a pure psychiatric presentation occurs in 20–25% of cases. Around 50% of patients will have mental disturbances at some point during the course of the disease. Psychiatric manifestations tend to occur more commonly with neurological forms of Wilson's disease than with the hepatic form of the clinical syndrome. Cognitive impairment occurs in up to 25% of patients. The dementia is usually subcortical type with frontal deficits. Depression occurs in 30% of cases and suicidal behaviour may occur in between 4 and 16%.

Ring HA, and Serra-Mestres J. Neuropsychiatry of the basal ganglia. *Journal of Neurology Neurosurgery and Psychiatry* 2002; **72**: 12–21.

102. E. It has been postulated that exposure of the brain to alcohol during the period of rapid synaptogenesis (third trimester) leads to apoptosis and neuronal loss, especially in thalamic and basal ganglia area. Since this change is apoptotic, it does not lead to fibrous scarring. This apoptotic cell death has been postulated to be due to the action of alcohol on the NMDA and GABA receptors. Apparently, large quantities of alcohol taken during a short period of time, even once, as in a binge episode, can lead to these changes. The cluster of symptoms also depends on the timing of alcohol exposure, so if the exposure occurred during the first trimester it would lead to facial abnormalities. In addition to developing hyperactivity/attention deficit disorder and varying degrees of learning impairment in children, a high percentage have adult-onset neuropsychiatric disturbances, including major depression and psychosis. There is no evidence to suggest that thiamine deficiency mediates neuronal damage in fetal alcohol syndrome.

Ramachandran VS, ed. *Encyclopedia of the Human Brain*, Vol. 1. Academic Press, 2002, p. 95–96.

103. C. Cauda equina syndrome is characterized by low back pain (radicular pain), asymmetric weakness, areflexia, and sensory loss in the legs, and relative sparing of bowel and bladder function. The syndrome usually results from injury of multiple lumbosacral nerve roots within the spinal canal. Most commonly, this is due to a ruptured lumbosacral intervertebral disc (disc prolapse). Less common causes include lumbosacral spine fracture, haematoma within the spinal canal, and compressive tumours. Cauda equine must be differentiated from conus medullaris syndrome, which includes compression of the lower sacral and coccygeal segments. This results in bilateral saddle anaesthesia, prominent bladder and bowel dysfunction, and impotence. Cutaneous reflexes are absent, but the muscle strength is usually preserved in conus medullaris syndrome.

Kasper DL *et al.*, eds. *Harrison's Principles of Internal Medicine*, 16th edn. McGraw-Hill, 2005, p. 98.

104. D. During embryonic development, gastrulation leads to the formation of the germ layers—ectoderm, mesoderm, and endoderm. Skin and nervous system develops from the ectoderm, the gut from the endoderm, and all other visceral organs from the mesoderm. After gastrulation, the notochord is formed from mesodermal cells. This notochord lies rostro caudally and it sends signals to the ectoderm lying adjacent to it, transforming them into neurectoderm. This forms the neuronal stem cells in the embryo. This strip of ectoderm is otherwise called the neuronal plate. By the third week of gestation, a groove develops on the dorsal aspect of the neural plate and this groove gradually deepens, forming neuronal folds. These folds gradually close bidirectionally by the end of the fourth week, forming the neural tube. Closure of the neural tube is susceptible to teratogenic influences operating in first trimester (e.g. valproate).

Ramachandran VS, ed. *Encyclopedia of the Human Brain*, Vol. 3. Academic Press, 2002, pp. 316–318.

105. E. Sphincter disturbance is not a feature of isolated cerebellar lesions. Unilateral lesions of the cerebellum affect ipsilateral limbs. Symptoms of cerebellar damage include asynergia (loss of coordination between muscles leading to jerky movements), dysmetria (defects in reaching targets via crude motor movements, for example past pointing on finger–nose test), intention tremor, dysarthria, disturbed balance including gait ataxia (produces wide-based, staggering gait prone to shuffle or fall), hypotonia, dysdiadochokinesia (inability to do rapid alternate movements), and nystagmus. The cerebellum has been suggested to be a seat of cognitive function, especially working memory.

Brazis P *et al. Localisation in Clinical Neurology*, 5th edn. Lippincott Williams and Wilkins, 2007, p. 372.

106. E. The vestibulocochlear nerve is purely sensory. It has two components, the vestibular and the cochlear, both of which are sensory. The vestibular component transmits information on position and balance received from the semicircular canals and the cochlear component serves the sense of hearing. The hypoglossal nerve innervates the ipsilateral side of the tongue. It is a purely motor efferent nerve. In unilateral lower motor neurone palsy of the eight nerve, when protruded, the tongue deviates toward the side of weakness. The trochlear nerve is unique among cranial nerves in that it decussates to the contralateral side and its point of exit is through the dorsal surface of the brain. The trochlear nerve thus innervates the superior oblique muscle of the contralateral eye. It is a purely efferent nerve. The facial nerve innervates the muscles of the face. It has a sensory component, innervating the anterior two-thirds of the tongue, via the chorda tympani. Facial nerve palsy causes deviation of the angle of mouth to the normal side. As a mnemonic, 'the rule of 17' applies to deviations in cranial nerve palsies. Palsy of tenth (vagus and hence palate) and seventh (facial) nerve leads to deviation to the normal side. Palsy of the fifth (trigeminal and hence the jaw muscles) and twelfth (hypoglossal, tongue) nerve leads to deviation to the paralytic side.

Ramachandran VS, ed. *Encyclopedia of the Human Brain*, Vol. 2. Academic Press, 2002, p. 65.

107. C. The pathway that enables normal vision starts from rods and cones in the retina, which are receptors of the ganglion cells. The axons of ganglion cells extend as the optic nerve, through the optic chiasma, via the optic tract, and synapse at the lateral geniculate body of thalamus. From the lateral geniculate body, second-order neurones go through the optic radiation to the visual cortex in the occipital lobe. In contrast, the pathway constituting the papillary light reflex digresses from the visual pathway before it joins the lateral geniculate body to reach the dorsal midbrain. They synapse at the pretectal nuclei, from where second-order neurones go to the Edinger–Westphal nucleus on both sides. Edinger–Westphal nuclei, via the third nerve, control the pupillary constrictors that constitute the response to light. So, pupillary light reflex do not involve the occipital cortex. Hence even in those with cortical blindness due to bilateral occipital cortex damage, light reflex may be intact.

Brazis P *et al. Localisation in Clinical Neurology*, 5th edn. Lippincott Williams & Wilkins, 2007, p. 158.

108. C. The hypoglossal nerve is a purely somatic motor nerve. The autonomic nervous system has two parts, the sympathetic and parasympathetic. Sympathetic output from the CNS is mainly through thoracic and lumbar spinal nerves. Sympathetic preganglionic nerves are short and form synapses in paired ganglia adjacent to the spinal cord. The parasympathetic system has a craniosacral output, that is it operates through some cranial nerves and sacral spinal nerves. These have long preganglionic nerves which form synapses at ganglia near or on the organ innervated. Among the cranial nerves, the vagus is the chief parasympathetic nerve. It supplies parasympathetic efferents to heart and most of the abdominal viscera and the gastrointestinal tract, but oculomotor (III), facial (VII), and glossopharyngeal nerves (IX) also carry parasympathetic fibres. The neurotransmitter at the preganglionic nerve ending is acetylcholine in both sympathetic and parasympathetic systems. At the post ganglionic nerve ending, the neurotransmitter is acetylcholine in the parasympathetic system and mostly norepinephrine in the sympathetic system.

Ramachandran VS, ed. *Encyclopedia of the Human Brain*, Vol. 2. Academic Press, 2002, p. 67.

109. D. The sympathetic system is responsible for the 'flight and fight' and the parasympathetic system for the 'rest and digest' reactions. Generally, they are considered to have opposing actions. The sympathetic system is activated in emergency situations, where the body requires more energy. This response includes increased cardiac output, dilatation of bronchioles, routing blood to the muscles, glycogen and fat breakdown leading to a rise in the blood glucose and fatty acids, and slowing down of digestion and renal filtration. This also leads to a decrease in gastrointestinal secretion and motility (leading to dryness of the mouth). In addition, sympathetic activity causes constriction of bladder and bowel sphincters and relaxation of the smooth muscles of the viscera. The pupils dilate due to action on the dilators. In contrast, parasympathetic stimulation leads to pupillary constriction and accommodation for close vision, reduces heart rate, constricts bronchioles, and increases gastrointestinal secretions with relaxation of sphincters. Parasympathetic stimulation is necessary for erection and sympathetic stimulation for ejaculation.

Ganong WF. *Review of Medical Physiology*, 22nd edn. McGraw-Hill, 2005, p. 229.

110. D. The posterior column is responsible for transmission of proprioception, light touch, tactile localization, and vibration senses. Posterior column dysfunction can result in disturbances in the knowledge of extremity movement and position. This presents as sensory ataxia (noted first in the dark as visual input does not compensate for the lost position sense) and a positive Romberg's sign. Pain and temperature is transmitted to the central nervous system through the spinothalamic tract. Spinothalamic tracts cross over two segments above the level of entry of the root at the spinal cord. Posterior column tracts cross over only at the midbrain level, where they synapse with the cuneate and gracilis nuclei. Hence, if hemisection of the cord takes place, ipsilateral posterior column senses are lost below the level of section; contralateral spinothalamic sensations are lost from two levels below the site of section.

Brazis P et al. Localization in Clinical Neurology, 5th edition. Lippincott Williams and Wilkins, 2006, p. 106.

111. A. The term basal ganglia traditionally applied to five large, subcortical nuclear masses on each side of the brain: the caudate nucleus, putamen, and globus pallidus, subthalamic nucleus, and substantia nigra. The globus pallidus is further divided into an external and an internal segment, and the substantia nigra is divided into a pars compacta and a pars reticulata. The caudate nucleus and the putamen are frequently called the striatum; the putamen and the globus pallidus are sometimes called the lenticular nucleus. The nucleus accumbens is the region where the putamen and the caudate merge anteriorly. What structures comprise the basal ganglia has been a debate over the years. More recently, an additional term, 'ventral striatum' has been introduced to describe those parts of the striatum (caudate and putamen) closest to limbic structures and that are involved in cognitive and behavioural functions. The ventral striatum includes the nucleus accumbens, which plays a major role in motivational and reward-related behaviour. Amygdala is closely related to the basal ganglia due to its functional and structural proximity. The amygdala complex develops from the same tissue mass as the caudate nucleus.

Ring HA and Serra-Mestres J. Neuropsychiatry of the basal ganglia. Journal of Neurology, Neurosurgery and Psychiatry 2002; **72**: 12– 21.

112. C. Horner's syndrome is caused by sympathetic dysfunction at the craniocervical output. Clinical features include ipsilateral mild (usually <2 mm) ptosis, anisocoria (unequal pupils) due to ipsilateral miosis, enophthalmos, loss of ciliospinal reflex, and ipsilateral facial anhidrosis (mnemonic 'PAMELA'). Nystagmus is generally not seen. Nystagmus is a rhythmical oscillation of the eyes, occurring pathologically in a wide variety of diseases. Abnormalities of the eyes or optic nerves, especially when the onset is in childhood, may present with nystagmus (pendular or jerk nystagmus). Jerk nystagmus is characterized by a slow drift off the target, followed by a fast corrective saccade. Jerk nystagmus can be downbeat, upbeat, or horizontal (left or right) with the names being given according to the direction of the fast phase. Gaze-evoked nystagmus is the most common form of jerk nystagmus, where the subject is asked to look to the corner of the eye. Exaggerated gaze-evoked nystagmus can be seen in: drug intake/toxicity (sedatives, anticonvulsants, alcohol); muscle paresis; myasthenia gravis; demyelinating disease; and cerebellopontine angle, brainstem, and cerebellar lesions. Downbeat nystagmus usually occurs from lesions near the craniocervical junction, while upbeat nystagmus is associated with damage to the pontine tegmentum, from stroke, demyelination, or tumour. Vestibular system dysfunction also leads to nystagmus. This occurs in discrete attacks, usually associated with sudden movements of the head and is accompanied by symptoms of nausea, tinnitus, hearing loss, and vertigo.

Kasper DL et al., eds. Harrison's Principles of Internal Medicine, 16th edn. McGraw-Hill, 2005, p. 176.

113. A. Ageing results in declines in a variety of cognitive domains, but some abilities appear to be relatively preserved. The relatively unaffected faculties include general intellectual knowledge, vocabulary and comprehension, attention processes, language abilities related to phonologic, lexical, and syntactic knowledge, motor skills that are learned early in life and repeatedly used, and immediate and implicit memory, including some aspects of short-term memory. Significant age-associated decline is seen in processing speed, ability to reason and solve problems, fluid intelligence, dividing attention between two tasks, executive function domains (mental flexibility, abstraction, and concept formation), visuospatial skills (drawing, construction, and maze learning), language skills involving semantic knowledge needed for naming and verbal fluency, motor skills that require speed, and ability to learn and retain new information for long-term access.

Ramachandran VS, ed. *Encyclopedia of the Human Brain*, Vol. 1. Academic Press, 2002, p. 48.

114. A. Gelastic seizures are characterized by shallow laughter occurring in fits. The laughter usually lasts less than 1 minute and is then followed by signs of complex partial or focal seizures, such as eye and head movement, automatisms such as lip-smacking, and altered awareness. In many cases, these associated features may be absent, resulting in delayed diagnosis. The most common areas of the brain associated with gelastic seizures are the hypothalamus, the temporal lobes, and the frontal lobes. A combination of gelastic seizures and precocious puberty is often noted and can be attributed to hamartoma of the hypothalamus.

Ropper AH and Brown RH, eds. *Adam and Victor's Principles of Neurology*, 8th edn. McGraw-Hill, 2005, p. 486.

115. C. The cholinergic nicotinic receptor forms the prototypical model for ionotropic receptors. It is a heteromeric pentameric protein, and each subunit is a transmembrane protein with four transmembrane domains (in total 20 transmembrane domains compared to seven in the case of metabotropic receptors). Binding of a neurotransmitter to the extracellular domain of the ionic receptor results in the brief opening of a transmembrane ionic pore. This leads to an influx of certain ions, which produces a brief modification of the resting membrane potential. This results in a postsynaptic action potential. Muscarinic acetyl choline receptors are not ionotropic; they are G-protein coupled and act via second messengers. $GABA_A$ not $GABA_B$ is an ion channel receptor. Norepinephrine receptors are largely G-protein coupled; they are not ion channels.

Ramachandran VS, ed. *Encyclopedia of the Human Brain*, Vol. 4. Academic Press, 2002, p. 525.

116. A. The presence of spiked red blood cells (RBCs) together with ataxia, progressive weakness, and cognitive impairment is suggestive of neuroacanthocytosis. Patients with neuroacanthocytosis may also show personality changes characterized by impulsivity, distractibility, and compulsivity. Neuropathological findings include severe atrophy of the caudate and putamen with loss of neurones and an associated astrocytic reaction. Less severe changes are seen in the pallidum, thalamus, substantia nigra, and anterior horn cells of spinal cord. Acanthocytes are spiked RBCs seen in peripheral blood smears. Acanthocytosis is also seen in patients with abetalipoproteinaemia or hypobetalipoproteinaemia, where serum vitamin E and lipoprotein levels are abnormal.

Ropper AH and Brown RH, eds. *Adam and Victor's Principles of Neurology*, 8th edn. McGraw-Hill, 2005, p. 913.

117. D.   The exact mechanisms of action of LSD and other hallucinogens are not completely understood as yet, but there is substantial evidence pointing towards serotonergic systems in the brain. Receptor-binding studies have shown that radiolabelled LSD binds to 5-HT$_{2A}$ and 5-HT$_{1C}$ receptors. Hallucinogens have agonist actions at the 5-HT$_{2A}$ receptor. The psychoactive and behavioural effects of hallucinogens are blocked by 5-HT$_{2A}$ antagonists. Tolerance/tachyphylaxis of hallucinogenic effect is related to down-regulation of 5-HT$_{2A}$ receptors. There may be a role for 5-HT$_{2C}$ receptors too in mediating the actions of hallucinogens. LSD is only a partial agonist at 5-HT$_{2A}$, in contrast to the full agonist actions of other hallucinogens. The 5-HT$_{2A}$ receptor potentiates glutamatergic and dopaminergic neurotransmission when activated, while activating the inhibitory GABA interneurone system.

Jakab RL and Goldman-Rakic PS. 5-Hydroxytryptamine2A serotonin receptors in the primate cerebral cortex: Possible site of action of hallucinogenic and antipsychotic drugs in pyramidal cell apical dendrites. *Proceedings of the National Academy of Sciences of the USA* 1998; **95**: 735–740. Kranzler HR and Ciraulo DA, eds. *Clinical Manual of Addiction Psychopharmacology*, 1st edn. American Psychiatric Publishing, 2005, p. 217.

118. B.   The acute administration of all addictive drugs (except benzodiazepines) stimulates dopamine transmission in the projection from the ventral mesencephalon to the nucleus accumbens. This projection is generally referred to as the mesolimbic dopamine system. The site of action by which different street drugs activate dopamine can be classified into three distinct types:
1. Increasing the presynaptic release of dopamine without directly altering the activity of dopamine neurones, for example stimulants acting via dopamine reuptake channels
2 Stimulation of dopamine neurones via receptors on dopaminergic neuronal membrane, for example marijuana via cannabinoid receptors
3. Via decrease of inhibitory input into dopaminergic cells leading to disinhibition of dopamine activity, for example opioids and alcohol.

Kay J and Tasman A. *Essentials of Psychiatry.* John Wiley and Sons, 2006, p. 150.

119. A.   Neurotrophins comprise a family of proteins including nerve growth factor (NGF), brain-derived neurotrophic factor (BDNF), and neurotrophins (NT)-3, -4/5, and -6. Proneurotrophins are enzymatically processed to create mature neurotrophins. Neurotrophins bind to specific tyrosine kinase receptors. Neurotrophins promote neuronal growth, differentiation, and survival, and modulate synaptic plasticity. These growth-related effects result from the interaction of neurotrophins with mitogen-activated protein kinase (MAPK) signalling pathway and the phosphatidylinositol-3 kinase pathway. In addition, the neurotrophins can inhibit cell death cascades. Reduced expression of neurotrophins such as BDNF has been proposed to underlie deficits in hippocampal neurogenesis seen in animal models of depression. Chronic antidepressant treatments are shown to upregulate neurotrophin expression, mediating relief from depression. Neurotrophin-mediated proliferation of hippocampal cells may be one of the final common pathways of antidepressant effects.

Fatemi HS and Clayton PJ. *Medical Basis of Psychiatry.* Humana Press, 2008, p. 524.

120. D. L-tyrosine is an amino acid derived from food proteins. It is also derived from the catabolism of phenylalanine in the liver by phenylalanine hydroxylase. L-tyrosine forms the precursor for the catecholamine neurotransmitters. Dopamine is the major initial product derived from L-tyrosine. Dopamine hydroxylase further converts dopamine into norepinephrine. In cells that contain phenylethanolamine N-methyltransferase (PNMT), norepinephrine undergoes further processing via methylation to produce epinephrine. Epinephrine is formed in trivial amounts in the CNS but is a major product in the adrenal medulla. Any drug that enhances the action of tyrosine hydroxylase and dopamine hydroxylase is likely to enhance noradrenergic transmission. Catecholamines are metabolized by two enzymes: monoamine oxidase (MAO) and catechol-O-methyl transferase (COMT).

Sadock BJ and Sadock VA. *Kaplan and Sadock's Synopsis of Psychiatry: Behavioral Sciences/Clinical Psychiatry*, 10th edn. Lippincott Williams and Wilkins, 2007, p. 103.

121. C. The majority of distributed serotonin in human body is located in the intestines. Due to the wide distribution of serotonin receptors, side-effects of serotonergic drugs may be variable; for example 5-HT$_3$ receptors in the area postrema or the hypothalamus are associated with nausea and vomiting. The receptors in the basal ganglia are associated with akathisia and agitation. Limbic receptors are associated with an anxiety response when serotonergic drugs are administered initially. The serotonin receptors in spinal cord may produce sexual dysfunction. The intestinal receptors constitute nearly 90% of the body's serotonin receptors. Hence the common side-effects with most serotonergic drugs are gastrointestinal upset and diarrhoea.

Sadock BJ and Sadock VA. *Kaplan and Sadock's Synopsis of Psychiatry: Behavioral Sciences/Clinical Psychiatry*, 10th edn. Lippincott Williams and Wilkins, 2007, p. 105.

122. E. The neurotransmitter that brings a signal to a neurone is considered to be the 'first messenger'. For the signal to get across to the postsynaptic neurone, it must be transformed into an intraneuronal message. This is enabled via formation of the 'second-messenger' molecules. Second messengers generally do not act outside the cell of origin. The most commonly encountered second messengers include cAMP and cGMP, the calcium ion (Ca^{2+}), and the phosphoinositol metabolites such as inositol triphosphate (IP3) and diacylglycerol (DAG). Gases such as nitric oxide and carbon monoxide also act as intraneuronal second-messenger molecules. The second messengers are not hormones as they do not reach tissues via the blood stream. Unlike receptor proteins, they do not combine with the neurotransmitter molecules directly. They are present throughout the CNS.

Sadock BJ and Sadock VA. *Kaplan and Sadock's Synopsis of Psychiatry: Behavioral Sciences/Clinical Psychiatry*, 10th edn. Lippincott Williams and Wilkins, 2007, p. 98.

123. A. This patient's presentation is suggestive of Bell's palsy. It is the most common cause of facial paralysis, usually occurring on one side only. The lifetime prevalence is about 1 in 60 in the UK. It is most commonly seen between the ages of 15 and 45, in both men and women. Pregnancy and diabetes may increase the risk of Bell's palsy substantially. Though the exact cause is not known, a viral aetiology is suspected (herpesvirus). The symptoms usually develop overnight. Most patients present with difficulty closing the eye, drooling of saliva, and sagging of the eyebrow on one side. Less commonly, patients may have heightened sensitivity to loud noise on the affected side. Most patients (nearly 80%) recover completely within 3 weeks. Almost all patients recover within 6 months. Patients with Bell's palsy exhibit Bell's phenomenon. Bell's phenomenon is a normal defence reflex present in about 75% of the population. It results in elevation of the globes when shutting eyes closed or when the eyes are directly threatened by external agents. Such upward movement helps to protect the most important structures (cornea and lens) of one's eyes. This elevation becomes noticeable when the orbicularis muscle becomes weak as in Bell's palsy. Bilateral Bell's phenomenon is found in myasthenia gravis, sarcoidosis, bilateral Bell's palsies, congenital facial diplegia, some rare forms of muscular dystrophy, motor neurone disease, and Guillain–Barré syndrome.

Holland NJ and Weiner GM. Recent developments in Bell's palsy. *British Medical Journal* 2004; **329**: 553–557.

124. C. Serotonergic cells are localized in the brainstem in a group of nuclei called the raphe nuclei. In contrast to the more circumscribed dopaminergic pathways, almost all parts of the brain receive serotonergic input. This probably explains the multiple effects of serotonin receptors on mood and behaviour. All serotonin receptors are G-protein linked, except 5-HT_3 which is ligand gated. Serotonin does not cross the blood–brain barrier and thus the brain synthesizes its own serotonin. This is in turn determined by concentrations of free plasma tryptophan and transport across the blood–brain barrier. This forms the basis of the rapid tryptophan depletion test. Tryptophan hydroxylase hydroxylates tryptophan to 5-hydroxy tryptophan (5-HTP), which is further decarboxylated to serotonin (5-HT) by aromatic-L-amino acid decarboxylase (AADC) in the presence of vitamin B_6 as coenzyme. The rate-limiting step in serotonin synthesis is considered to be the availability of 5-HTP. In parallel with dopamine and norepinephrine, following release into the synaptic cleft, 5-HT is either metabolized or actively transported back into the neurone by a high-affinity transporter, the serotonin reuptake transporter (SERT). SERT is encoded by a single gene on chromosome 17. The SERT gene has been recently postulated to play an important role in gene–environment interaction in disorders such as depression.

Gillette R. Evolution and function in serotonergic systems. *Integrative and Comparative Biology* 2006; **46**: 838–846.

Caspi A, Sugden K, Moffitt TE *et al.* Influence of life stress on depression: Moderation by a polymorphism in the 5-HTT gene. *Science* 2003; **301**: 386–389.

125. C. Prion protein (PrP) is a glycoprotein anchored to neuronal cell membranes. The normal function of prion protein is not known. Bovine spongiform encephalopathy ('mad cow disease') and Crutzfeldt–Jakob disease are associated with altered prion proteins. In prion diseases, the normal cellular form of PrP (called PrP^C) undergoes transformation to an altered version (called scrapie-associated prion protein PrP^{Sc}). The latter accumulates in the brain to form insoluble aggregates, leading to neuronal dysfunction, but unlike other neurodegenerative diseases, prion diseases are transmissible. This is made possible because PrP^{Sc} imprints its pathological conformation onto other, normal PrP^C molecules, thus 'converting' them to be abnormal. PrP^C and PrP^{Sc} do not differ in their amino acid sequences.

Aguzzi A, Baumann F, and Bremer J. The prion's elusive reason for being. *Annual Review of Neuroscience* 2008; **31**: 439–477.

126. D. The establishment and maintenance of a wakeful state is called arousal. In humans, arousal activity requires at least three brain regions. The most important of these is the ascending reticular activating system (ARAS). ARAS may have a role in setting the level of consciousness. ARAS, via the intralaminar nuclei of the thalamus, project widely throughout the cerebral cortex. A synchronized, rhythmic burst of neuronal activity (20–40 Hz frequency) results from ARAS and thalamic coordination. The degree of synchronization varies directly with the level of wakefulness. During sleep the synchronicity is lost. The third most important region in arousal state is the right frontal lobe. The right frontal lobe is essential for the 'maintenance' of attention; this is evident when testing letter-cancellation tasks or trail-making tasks in patients with right frontal lesions.

Sadock BJ and Sadock VA. *Kaplan and Sadock's Synopsis of Psychiatry: Behavioral Sciences/Clinical Psychiatry*, 10th edn. Lippincott Williams and Wilkins, 2007, p. 87.

127. E. Hodgkin and Huxley showed that the inside of a cell, such as a neurone, is negatively charged compared to the outside. This is called the resting membrane potential and its value ranges between −40 mV and −90 mV (average −70 mV), depending on the type of cell. This negative resting membrane potential arises due to the membranes of the resting neurone being more permeable to potassium ions than to any other ions. There are more potassium ions inside the cell than outside it, which is due to a constant outward leak creating a negative potential inside the cell. An action potential is initiated in the axon hillock when the synaptic signals received by the dendrites and soma are sufficient to raise the intracellular potential from −70 mV to the threshold potential of −55 mV. When this potential is reached, the Na^+ channels, which are dormant at rest, will open. This Na^+ influx causes rapid reversal of the membrane potential from −70 to +40 mV.

Ramachandran VS, ed. *Encyclopedia of the Human Brain*, Vol. 1. Academic Press, 2002, p. 1–12.

128. D. Glycine is an inhibitory transmitter, predominantly found in the spinal cord; it has relatively insignificant effects in the brain compared to the spinal cord. Glycine acts on a chloride channel that is different from $GABA_A$ receptors, called the strychnine-sensitive glycine receptor. On activation, the transmembrane glycine receptors facilitate entry of chloride ion into the cell, leading to hyperpolarization of the cell. Glycine is synthesized from serine; this conversion is mediated by rate-limiting steps via serine trans-hydroxymethylase and glycerate dehydrogenase. Glycine also serves as an obligatory neurotransmitter adjunct for glutamate activity on the NMDA glutamate receptors (non-strychnine-sensitive glycine site). Some clinical trials have shown a reduction in the negative symptoms of schizophrenia using D-serine or glycine mediated via NMDA receptors, though this has not been widely replicated.

Sadock BJ and Sadock VA. *Kaplan and Sadock's Synopsis of Psychiatry: Behavioral Sciences/Clinical Psychiatry*, 10th edn. Lippincott Williams and Wilkins, 2007, p. 109.

129. C. Positron emission tomography (PET) is considered as the gold standard of functional neuroimaging modalities. Among other available techniques, only PET can measure cerebral glucose metabolism directly. In addition, a large number of radioligands for receptor characterization are available for PET. Despite these advantages, PET is not widely available due to the expensive nature of the equipment; it requires relatively rapid access to a cyclotron to produce the positron-emitting radionuclides.

Kay J and Tasman A. *Essentials of Psychiatry*. John Wiley and Sons, 2006, p. 232.

130. C. Most hormones show a diurnal–nocturnal variation in their plasma levels. This is partly related to circadian mechanisms and hypothalamic functions. Level of physical activity and diurnal change in metabolic requirements may also influence the hormonal levels in blood. Growth hormone regulates carbohydrate and lipid metabolism. There is a nocturnal surge of growth hormone seen during slow wave sleep (stage 3 and 4 NREM sleep). Speculative association of growth hormone surge and memory consolidation has not been borne out by experimental results.

Gais S, Hüllemann P, Hallschmid M *et al.* Sleep-dependent surges in growth hormone do not contribute to sleep-dependent memory consolidation. *Psychoneuroendocrinology* 2006; **31**: 786–791.

131. C. The presentation here is consistent with craniopharyngioma. It is a benign, slow-growing tumour involving the pituitary gland. The clinical presentation is usually insidious with the most common presenting symptoms being headache, endocrine dysfunction, and visual field disturbances. The headache may be positional and slowly progressive. Hypothyroidism, adrenal failure, and diabetes insipidus are the common endocrine disturbances noted. Young patients may have growth failure and/or delayed puberty. Visual field defects are due to pressure effects on the optic nerve route. Bitemporal hemianopia is the most common problem due to pressure at the chiasma. The anatomic location of the craniopharyngioma may be classified into prechiasmal (associated with optic atrophy), retrochiasmal (associated with signs of increased intracranial pressure such as papilledema), or intrasellar (associated with headache and endocrine dysfunction). The diagnosis is strongly suggested by imaging studies. The appearance of a suprasellar or intrasellar calcified cyst is considered to be the radiological hallmark. CT scan is the most sensitive method as calcifications are easily picked up as high-density areas. MRI is very helpful for neurosurgeons to plan a surgical approach.

Ropper AH and Brown RH, eds. *Adams and Victor's Principles of Neurology*, 8th edn. McGraw-Hill, 2005, pp. 573–574.

132. E. The embryogenetic theory of craniopharyngioma suggests the involvement of Rathke's pouch. The infundibulum is a downward projection of diencephalon; the Rathke's pouch is an upward elongation of the primitive oral cavity. Rathke's pouch and the infundibulum develop during the fourth week of gestation and grow towards each other until they unite to form the hypophysis of the pituitary gland during the second month. The remnants of Rathke's pouch involute into a cleft and disappear completely in normal conditions. In some cases, this Rathke's cleft remnant can become the site of origin of craniopharyngiomas. Alar plate is related to development of the spinal cord. Isthumus of thyroid is related to thyroglossal duct.

Ropper AH and Brown RH, eds. *Adams and Victor's Principles of Neurology*, 8th edn. McGraw-Hill, 2005, pp. 573–574.

133. D. The patient described in Question 133 has an acute onset of flinging movements of one side of the body. This is called hemiballism. Movements are usually involuntary, wide amplitude, and irregular with no pattern or rhythm. They commonly involve the arm and leg together; facial involvement has been reported in about half of the cases. Movements are increased with action, decreased with relaxation, and absent during sleep. In some patients the movements can cause physical exhaustion or injury of the affected limb. Hemiballism is considered to be primarily a disorder of the contralateral subthalamic nuclei (STN), but recently lesions outside STN have been demonstrated in patients with hemiballism. It is noted that the hemiballism caused by lesions of the STN is more severe than that caused by lesions elsewhere.

Posturna RB and Lang AE. Hemiballism: revisiting a classic disorder. *Lancet Neurology* 2003; **2**: 661–668.

134. C. The cardinal function of prefrontal cortex is planning and organization of behaviour (executive function) in addition to functions of short-term memory, motor attention, and inhibitory control. The change in Gage's personality would be consistent with damage to the orbitofrontal cortex of the ventral aspect of his frontal lobe, affecting affect and emotion. A pseudopsychopathic syndrome, characterized by impulsivity and socially inappropriate behaviour, is recognized in orbitofrontal damage. Inferior parietal cortex may play a role in attention and body image function. The primary function of superior temporal cortex is auditory processing. The hippocampus is the seat of episodic memory; lesions can result in amnesia. The hypothalamus is involved in appetitive behaviours such as hunger, thirst, and sex.

O'driscoll K and Leach JP. 'No longer Gage': an iron bar through the head. *British Medical Journal* 1998; **317**: 1673–1674.

135. A. Mononeuritis multiplex is a form of peripheral neuropathy wherein axonal destruction occurs in different sites leading to sensory and motor deficits. The nerves involved are generally multiple and random with no predictability of progression. This acute or subacute involvement of multiple individual nerves may be serial or even simultaneous. It is not a single disease but a syndrome caused by various disorders; often the final common pathway includes vascular damage to neurones. Nearly one-third of cases are idiopathic. The most common identifiable cause in adults is diabetes mellitus, followed by vasculitis syndromes such as polyarteritis nodosa and connective tissue diseases such as rheumatoid arthritis or systemic lupus erythematosus. In children and adolescents, the most common cause of mononeuritis multiplex is connective tissue disease. Mononeuritis multiplex can mimic conversion disorder and present to psychiatric units.

Ropper AH and Brown RH, eds. *Adams and Victor's Principles of Neurology*, 8th edn. McGraw-Hill, 2005, p. 1137.

136. E. The question describes the classic form of the Stroop Colour–Word Test. In this test the subject is initially required to read names of some basic colours. Later the subject is asked to name the colours of geometrical shapes. Following this, the test of interference is applied. Looking at a colour name written in a different colour produces a conflict; this makes the subject read the name instead of saying the colour in which it is written, for example if the word 'blue' is written in green the subject tends to say blue, even when asked to name the displayed colour. The classic form of the Stroop Colour–Word Test is the most commonly used, though variations such as Emotional Stroop are now available. Rorschach's is a projective test which uses ink-blot images. The Continuous Performance Test measures sustained/selective attention and impulsivity.

Goldfarb L and Henik A. New data analysis of the stroop matching task calls for a reevaluation of theory. *Psychological Science* 2006; **17**: 96–100.

137. A. Dopamine is synthesized from the amino acid tyrosine. Initially, tyrosine is converted to L-dihydroxyphenylalanine (L-DOPA) by tyrosine hydroxylase (the rate-limiting step). L-DOPA is rapidly converted to dopamine by dopa decarboxylase. Dopamine is stored in vesicles and 80% of the released dopamine is rapidly transported back into the nerve terminal by a dopamine-specific transporter (DAT). This intracellular extravesicular dopamine is metabolized by monoamine oxidase (MAO) to dihydroxyphenylacetic acid (DOPAC). Twenty percent of the released dopamine is sequentially degraded extracellularly by catechol-O-methyltransferase (COMT) and MAO to 3-methoxytyramine (3-MT) and homovanillic acid (HVA). Dopaminergic cell bodies in the brain are mainly localized in the ventral tegmental area in the brainstem. There are predominantly four pathways that are considered to be dopaminergic in the brain: mesocortical and mesolimbic axons originate from the VTA and project to the prefrontal cortex and limbic structures, respectively; the tuberoinfundibular pathway mediates release of prolactin from the pituitary; and the nigrostriate pathway forms an integral part of the basal ganglion extrapyramidal system.

Elsworth JD and Roth RH. Dopamine synthesis, uptake, metabolism, and receptors: relevance to gene therapy of Parkinson's disease. *Experimental Neurology* 1997; **144**: 4–9.

138. C. Parkinsonian tremor is usually of large amplitude with a frequency of 4 to 6 cycles per second. It is a resting tremor which persists even during action. Parkinsonian tremor is not reduced by alcohol but is exaggerated in stressful situations. In contrast, benign essential tremor is usually of smaller amplitude and higher frequency (10 to 12 cycles per second). It is often seen during action and may be unnoticeable during rest. It is exacerbated by stress, similar to Parkinsonian tremor. Clinically, essential tremor is similar to exaggerated physiological tremor.

Cummings JL and Trimble M. *Neuropsychiatry and Behavioural Neurology.* American Psychiatric Publishing, 2002, p. 187.

139. D. The patient described here has acute, severe headache, photophobia, and meningism. These features are highly suggestive of subarachnoid haemorrhage (SAH). A CT scan is not 100% sensitive in ruling out possible intracranial bleed. Given the high clinical suspicion, the gold standard test for SAH, lumbar puncture, must be carried out. Presence of depression must not distract one from considering acute medical causes of somatic complaints such as headaches. Haloperidol is not indicated in this scenario. Please note that if the CT scan discloses a subarachnoid haemorrhage, lumbar puncture need not be carried out as a routine.

Ropper AH and Brown RH, eds. *Adams and Victor's Principles of Neurology*, 8th edn. McGraw-Hill, 2005, p. 328.

140. C. This patient is having an infarct of the thalamus. Thalamic infarcts affecting ventral posterolateral nucleus and posteromedial nucleus result in a severe sensory syndrome characterized by intense burning pain, hyperaesthesia, or hemianaesthesia affecting the contralateral body. Cold thermal stimuli, emotional stress, and loud sounds may aggravate the painful state. Despite this apparent hypersensitivity, the patient shows an elevated pain threshold requiring a stronger than usual stimulus to produce a sensation of pain (hypoalgesia with hyperpathia). This thalamic pain syndrome is also called Dejerine–Roussy syndrome. Some patients may develop hemiataxia and choreoathetosis.

Ropper AH and Brown RH, eds. *Adams and Victor's Principles of Neurology*, 8th edn. McGraw-Hill, 2005, p. 141.

Key: ■ denotes question, ■ denotes answer